If I Love You,
Why Is It So Hard to Live With You?

Learning How to Create a Healthy Intimate Relationship

By Susan Gleeson, M.D.

Copyright © 2013 by Susan Gleeson

Published by Lulu.com

ISBN: 978-1-304-31552-6

For Alannah,
because I promised
I would write this book for you.

For Laura,
for giving me the idea for the book's title.

For Dad,
because you always believed in me.
Allan Joseph Gleeson
(October 30, 1928 - October 19, 2012)

ACKNOWLEDGMENTS

It takes many people to accomplish the goal of writing and publishing a book. I am blessed to have a wonderful editor, Joan Williams, a Lulu navigator extraordinaire, Sheri Smith, a gifted and patient book cover designer, Lee Xu, and many willing friends who acted as readers of various parts of the manuscript in service of writing a book that would be as accurate, honest, clear, and helpful as possible for you, the reader.

For all those who helped make this book, I am deeply grateful. I could not have done it without you!

If I Love You, Why Is It So Hard to Live With You?
Learning How to Create a Healthy Intimate Relationship

TABLE OF CONTENTS

A troubled woman sat across from me in my coaching room and began to speak. *"I feel like I am sinking deeper and deeper into a dark, bottomless hole. I am feeling more and more lost and alone, but I don't know why. I have a kind husband, a good job and children who I adore, yet somehow I feel that everything in my life is going wrong. My husband is a good man, but every time I try to explain why I feel miserable, I just can't get him to understand. I've begun to resent him. I don't know whether the problem is me, my job or my marriage, or if it could be a combination of all of them. I have been putting a lot of energy into our relationship but it's not helping. I just keep falling deeper into that black hole. Do you think you can help me understand myself and my relationship? Do you think I can ever be contented again?"*

In the past decade as a life coach, I have worked with many individuals who feel as despondent as this person. I have also met people just like her during the course of my day-to-day medical practice of 30 years—people who appear, from the outside, to have it all together, but who are actually feeling intense despair.

I call this situation Soul Misery because the condition of apparently having it all yet feeling empty and rudderless can produce a state of deep suffering. This suffering is felt in a place within us that is somehow different than the mind or the heart. This suffering is felt deep within our core, within that place we call our soul.

In my first book, *Healing Soul Misery: Finding the Pathway Home,* I began by asking clients to describe how Soul Misery felt for them. One sufferer described a bleak day-to-day experience.

"It's a state of desperation, without much hope for change to occur. It is confusion. It is a yearning to discover where the pain is really coming from. It's feeling like giving up. The world has no colour. There's emotion, but no passion. There's existence, but no sense of light. Every once in a while, however, there is a spark—enough to keep seeking."

In addition to the confusion and pain, sufferers often feel they can't discover who they are or why they are here. Some reported feeling cut off from other people and, indeed, themselves. *"It's about feeling disconnected and isolated. It's never feeling authentic, doing what others want you to do, and not even knowing what you want to do."* Soul Misery probably sounds like depression to many people, yet it is not depression, although Soul Misery—if allowed to go on too long—can slip into a depression that co-exists with this condition.

Depression has classic signs and symptoms, such as difficulty with sleep, a lack of interest in life, strong feelings of guilt where it is not warranted, decreased energy, poor concentration, alterations of appetite, and decreased sexual interest. I have seen many people with personal Soul Misery who had none of these signs and symptoms, and who, in fact, were highly functioning members of society.

Soul Misery is a more existential experience because the person is searching deeply for the meaning in their life; they desperately need to know what it is. It regards knowing clearly who they are and why they are here, as well as having someone else see it, too. Exquisite pain can accompany the awareness that no one else can see clearly *who I am.* There is neither the sense of deep in-the-belly contentment that arises from really knowing oneself, nor the joy and relief of being truly seen by another.

In my first book, I discussed what causes personal Soul Misery. I described the four stages of healing from the standpoint of the individual who is suffering this condition. Although Soul Misery *is* a grim and dark situation, the good news is that Soul Misery can be alleviated. There is, indeed, a way to find the pathway home to ourselves. In this book, I want to discuss Soul Misery in the context of an intimate relationship. Soul Misery in Relationship is a more complex topic, because we must take into account not only what is going on inside of us, but also what is going on inside our intimate partner, as well as what is happening within the unique entity that is formed by the two of us together. In my experience, Soul Misery in Relationship always co-exists with personal Soul Misery in one of the partners. One partner is suffering personal Soul Misery, trying to make sense of it and battle their way out. Often that partner doesn't know the origin of their Soul Misery, as in the case of the woman we heard from first--sitting in the coaching room and feeling terribly lost. She just knows she is suffering greatly and is very puzzled that somehow her spouse is not able to understand or provide her with any help or consolation. She is feeling utterly alone with her pain.

Of course, at their best, committed, long-term, intimate relationships provide us a safe and secure lifelong place of belonging, companionship, comfort, and joy. However, for people trying to make sense of--and heal--their personal Soul Misery, their attempts to learn about who they are and become who they were born to be can place them for the first time in opposition to the very person from whom they received love and a sense of belonging. Soul Misery sufferers are going through a deep process of transformation, and they find to their chagrin that the one closest to them may not like it or even understand it at all, especially because it may threaten the comfortable, former status quo of the relationship. They may find themselves asking questions such as, *Will my partner still be able to love the person I am becoming? Will the person I am becoming still feel love for my partner?* These are frightening questions! As these individuals grow and change, they begin to wonder if it is going to be possible to relate effectively enough to meet both their need—and their partner's need–for love and approval and belonging.

As you begin to read this book, perhaps you feel that you are experiencing Soul Misery in your relationship, or you know someone who is, or maybe you have left a relationship due to Soul Misery. Perhaps you are simply attracted by the title of this book and want to learn more about how to create a healthy intimate relationship. No matter how you are feeling about being in a relationship right now, or what stage you may be at in the life of your partnership—beginning, middle, or end—it is entirely possible to gain additional information, learn new behaviours, and come from more powerful perspectives that will help you feel happier and function more effectively. In *If I Love You, Why Is It So Hard to Live With You?* it is my goal, my task, and my joy to provide a practical toolkit that I believe will help give you a new sense of competence and satisfaction in your intimate relationship.

What are the thoughts and feelings of individuals who take that first brave step toward understanding the unrest they feel within themselves and within their relationships? I asked people suffering what I have come to call Soul Misery in Intimate Relationship to define this uneasy condition for me. The overriding feeling among most of them was a lack of emotional connection with their partner.

"Soul misery in my marriage felt like I was suffocating, as if oxygen was not flowing easily. STUCK! It was, at times, a great challenge to find the beauty and miracles all around me when I was feeling that level of a void... The deal-breaker for me was not being able to feel connected on an emotional level after so many years of trying."

"It's scary to think that I could have committed to being with someone who really didn't 'get me' and with whom I couldn't have a two-way talk about things that made my heart sing."

"I have experienced Soul Misery in my relationship as a lack of conversational rhythm when interacting either one-on-one, or when we're together in social settings."

Not enjoying meaningful conversation makes Soul Misery in Intimate Relationship feel like you are very alone. There is no one to mirror back to you what you have said to show you have been deeply heard and understood, which is one of the great joys of being in a companionable relationship. One client reported feeling so disheartened that he felt himself beginning to shut down. *"Not feeling seen or heard beyond the surface content of my words muzzles my spirit, as though I were in captivity."*

Some individuals define Soul Misery in Intimate Relationship as feeling confused; they cannot figure out what is wrong in a relationship that used to feel so close and fulfilling. *"Early on, my marriage felt quite satisfying. We shared common values and a common faith. We were a good parenting team. However, after our children reached their teenage years, I began to feel a void-- and what was worse--I didn't know where that void was coming from. My partner was still the same good person. I was, too. What was going wrong for us?"*

And then there are clients who experienced Soul Misery in marriage as feeling hopeless, so hopeless, in fact, that they entertained a desire to flee the relationship. *"When I took my vows, they were for better, for worse, for richer or poorer, until death do us part. I meant them at the time and I wanted to continue to honour them. But it began to feel impossible. I thought I would rather live alone than live this way--with the sadness of not feeling deeply seen and deeply understood. I didn't understand why this mattered now so deeply to me, whereas it didn't before. Nonetheless, the feelings were so intense, I just wanted to escape."*

Reading these definitions show us that Soul Misery in Intimate Relationship can be an acutely painful state. We can feel confused, lost, alone, hopeless, empty, and desperately unhappy. We may feel as if we can't stand it any longer. We wonder how we can possibly be who we are and at the same time find a way to belong within the relationship that matters so much to us.

In order to both be *and* belong we need to understand as deeply as possible how we *tick* as individuals and then live in accordance with what we discover. We also need to learn as much as possible about the personality, values, needs, and wants of the people we love. And we need to become students of how relationships work in general, and in turn, study the workings of our own unique partnership. Our relationships are like a dance and each relationship steps and sways in a dance unique to its own beat. We can learn to appreciate, and to love, the secrets and the mysteries of our one-of-a-kind relationship.

I believe that knowledge of self + knowledge of our loved one + strong relationship skills give us the best possible chance at a successful union. Three things come together to determine how we feel about the health of our relationship.

Me = how I am being in my life and how that impacts You

You = who You are being and what I expect and assume of You

We/Our Relationship = how We actually relate together

Come with me, and we will begin the process of learning much more about *Me, You,* and *We.*

CHAPTER ONE   Me:
                    In Order To Love Another
              I Must Be in the Process of Becoming a Whole Person

A dynamic relationship is made up of two complete individuals
who respect each other's boundaries.

> Geoff Charley and Lucy Lidell
> *The Mirror Cards: A Powerful Tool to Enhance Your*
> *Relationship*

Let us begin by putting aside, for the time being, the many
thoughts, concerns, and feelings we may have about our partner.
Instead, let us take a journey inward and see what we find there.
A good place to start this exhilarating journey is to ask ourselves,
what does it mean to be *a "complete" individual*?

I believe a complete individual is someone who is aware of who
they are and who they are designed to be. I also believe that each
person has been individually designed to fulfil a purpose unique
to them. We all have specific physical characteristics, a
personality type, gifts, talents, and abilities that fit us for the
unique purpose for which we were made--our original design.
The more we know about who we are and who we were designed
to be, the more complete we are and the more complete we feel.

A colleague of mine put it this way: *"Being 'complete' implies
the absence of Soul Misery. It's having a clear sense of purpose
and worth in the world. That individual understands their own
needs and has developed the capacity to get their needs met. It
implies some mastery of navigating the world, understanding
what they need and knowing how to get it for themselves."*

Helping people discover their sense of purpose--who they are and why they are here--is the most important work I do as a life coach. When we know these things about ourselves, our lives begin to make sense. We develop a clear inner guidance system. As we begin to make life choices based on knowing who we are and why we are here, our judgement regarding those choices improves.

In his book *Finding Meaning in the Second Half of Life: How to Finally Really Grow Up*, Jungian analyst James Hollis gives us a term for this process: *individuation*. Individuation in its psychological sense is a concept first developed by the psychiatrist Carl Jung. Many writers have expounded on Jung's idea, Hollis among them. Hollis believes individuation requires from us a lasting commitment.

> Individuation is the life-long project of becoming more nearly the whole person we were meant to be--what the gods intended, not the parents, or the tribe, or, especially, the easily intimidated or inflated ego... So often the idea of individuation has been confused with self-indulgence or mere individualism, but what individuation more often asks of us is the surrender of the ego's agenda of security and emotional reinforcement, in favour of humbling service to the soul's intent. (Hollis 10)

Daring to desire to discover all of who we are and what we are destined to be in the world--and then to pursue it--can be frightening. Scholar Joseph Campbell referred to the process as "the hero's journey." In *Reflections on the Art of Living: A Joseph Campbell Companion*, Diane Osbon compares embarking on the hero's journey to stepping over a threshold.

There *is* a track just waiting there for each of us, and
once on it, doors will open that were not open before
and would not open for anyone else… The heroic first
step of the journey is out of, or over the edge of, your
boundaries, and is often taken before you know that
you will be supported. The hero's journey has been
compared to a birth: it starts with being warm and snug
in a safe place; then comes a signal, growing more
insistent, that it is time to leave. (9, 10)

It can be easier to become who our parents, our teachers, or other
authority figures say we should be and to fit into society as a
good citizen and respectable group member. But one of the
rewards inherent in travelling the road to become more and more
the whole person we were intended to be, is that we are then
fitted to function as a healthy, conscious person in a relationship.
I believe when we feel whole, we are more able and willing to
take responsibility to know and meet our own needs, rather than
requiring our intimate partner to meet them. And this is very
good for the relationship, as it takes the pressure off our partner
to feel obliged in some way to do tasks and meet needs for us that
are actually ours to accomplish. How do we begin the journey of
discovering this whole person we are intended to be? A valuable
start is to realize just how influenced we are by those around us--
their values, and their ideas of how we should live our lives.

Domestication: Who Was I Socialized To Be?

In my book *Healing Soul Misery: Finding the Pathway Home,* I discuss in detail the process that writer Don Miguel Ruiz terms "domestication." In his book, *The Four Agreements,* Ruiz says when we are born we become subject to what he terms the "dream of the planet."

> The dream of the planet includes all of society's rules, its beliefs, its laws, its religions, its different cultures, and ways to be, its governments, schools, social events, and holidays. We are born with the capacity to learn how to dream and the humans who live before us teach us how to dream the way society dreams. The outside dream has so many rules that when a new human is born we hook the child's attention and introduce these rules into his or her mind. The outside dream uses Mom and Dad, the schools, and religions to teach us how to dream. (2-3)

In other words, in North American society, parents usually tend to prioritise socializing a newborn child according to the rules of society, rather than focusing on the uniqueness of their child and trying to draw out and encourage that uniqueness. Parents seek to mold a child to be a good citizen within the family and within the society, and rightly so, for the good of society. However, I believe an equally important task for parents is to look deeply for the inherent gifts, talents, and abilities of their son or daughter as they surface (his or her original design) and then to encourage those unique attributes. Teachers, ministers--even aunts and uncles--in addition to promoting the behaviours of a good group member, could consciously choose to be equally concerned with seeking out and encouraging the original design of each child.

Good citizens are crucial to a functioning society, but because domestication is usually the focus of childrearing, it is not surprising that children can grow into adults who do not know themselves deeply. When we do not know who we are, we cannot be the whole, complete, happy, contented, fulfilled person we want and need to be to function as good partners in a relationship. Also, when we know who we are and "how we tick," we will be in a better position to choose a partner who is the best possible fit with who we are and what we need in a relationship.

Myers Briggs Personality Typing: Who Am I?

There are many methods of self-discovery, but the one I have found most helpful as a starting point in the journey to wholeness is the Myers-Briggs personality typing system. As I discussed in *Healing Soul Misery: Finding the Pathway Home,* two Americans, Kathryn Briggs and her daughter, Isabel Briggs Myers became so fascinated by Carl Jung's book *Psychological Types* that they went on to study Jung's work in detail (40). These women expanded Jung's findings and developed the Myers Briggs Type Indicator Test (MBTI), which is a detailed document designed to measure psychological type.

Jung documented three personality preferences and eight personality types. Myers and Briggs, based on their many years of study, identified four personality preferences and sixteen distinct personality types.

Instead of describing her sixteen types in a narrative, Myers elected to label each one with a kind of shorthand. She combined single letters chosen from four pairs of alternatives, E or I, S or N, T or F, J or P. Each letter represents the following psychological characteristic:

❖ E = Extraverted   or   I = Introverted

❖ S = Sensory   or   N = Intuitive

❖ T = Thinking   or   F = Feeling

❖ J = Judging   or   P = Perceiving

- Myers described being extraverted as having an "expressive" and outgoing social attitude.
- Introverted means having a "reserved" and reclusive attitude.
- Sensory means being highly "observant" of things in the immediate environment.
- Intuitive means being "introspective" or highly imaginative of things seen only with the mind's eye.
- Thinking means being "tough minded" or objective and impersonal with others.
- Feeling means being "friendly" or sympathetic and personal with others.
- Judging means being given to making and keeping schedules.
- Perceiving means looking around for alternatives, opportunities and options, hence probing or exploring. (Keirsey, *Please Understand Me ll*, 12-13)

As a life coach, one of the first exercises I do with a client is to help them ascertain their own personality type in relation to these variables. Using the method described in the book *Do What You Are* by Paul Tieger and Barbara Barron-Tieger, we begin the process of deciding which combination of the four letters best fit my client. It is an interesting process for each person, and--almost always--is fairly easy for the client to determine. When we ascertain their personality type, reading the more detailed description of that type proves invaluable, as the client will usually laugh out loud and say, *how can they possibly know me that well?* They are delighted to discover something this basic and this important about themselves.

I find that, as most people are unaware of their personality type, it follows that many are not living in conjunction with their personality type. If we are not *living out* who we are, we will be confused, unsatisfied, and certainly not feeling whole, happy, and free. How does this happen to us?

First of all, most parents are unaware that there are 16 different and distinct personality types, each of which has important functions in society and all of which have just as much right as another to exist. Of course, we will tend to view ways of being or behaving that are the same as our own as "normal." So a person who is, for example, an ESTJ (Extroverted Sensor Thinking Judging) personality who is parenting an INFP (Introverted Intuitive Feeling Perceiver) child will tend to encourage extraverted(E), concrete(S), logical and analytical(T), scheduled (J) behaviour, because--for them--this seems "normal." Moreover, as Tieger and Barron-Tieger estimate the ESTJ personality type as representing approximately 12-15% of the (American) population, the ESTJ parent can look around and find many mirrors--or reflections--of himself or herself, which further supports their belief that their way of being in the world is, in fact, "normal" (Tieger and Barron-Tieger 43).

This style of parenting, however, can cause turmoil, confusion, and pain for an INFP child. (Although gender plays no part in Meyers-Briggs typing, for this example I will use a female child.) This INFP child's natural inclination is to be reclusive, desiring a lot of quiet time alone (I). She has an introspective nature and looks inside herself rather than to the external world to find inspiration (N). She is a child who feels deeply(F) and she feels happiest leaving her options open (P). If her natural tendencies are not reinforced by her parents, and she is encouraged to behave in ways contrary to her nature, she can feel deeply unhappy *and have no idea why.* This produces Soul Misery--the state of not knowing who she is, not knowing why she doesn't feel right inside, and feeling unaccountably upset. She feels like an ugly duckling in her family, when in fact, she may be a chickadee born into a duck family! To make matters worse, as the INFP personality type only represents 3-4% of the (American) population, the ESTJ parent may not recognize their child's personality type if they do not have friends or family members of the INFP type (37).

Tieger and Barron-Tieger also have written a book called *Nurture by Nature* that teaches parents how to recognize their children's personality type and how to nurture that child in the way she or he uniquely needs to be nurtured. If more of us had the experience of being raised by parents who were either similar to us in personality type, or who were aware of the fact that there are 16 different, unique, equally worthy personality types, fewer people would experience Soul Misery; more of us would be living in accordance with our innate personality type.

Knowing which personality type we are and *living* it enhances our ability to enjoy more positive intimate relationships. We show up as we are, rather than appearing as the person we have been domesticated to be. When this is the case, a prospective partner can actually see who we are and choose to engage in a relationship based on us being a true representation of who we are. Even if we didn't have parents to help us identify our true nature, it's never too late to learn about ourselves in this way and bring this new self-knowledge to our relationships.

Personal Values: What Do I Value and What Brings Meaning to My Life?

My next step in helping a client on their journey of self-discovery is to help them discover their personal values. Values are simply the things that we value in life, the principles and ideas that are intrinsically desirable and important in our lives. I believe that a person's values are inborn, distinctive to that individual alone and part of our original design. I have worked with hundreds of clients and I have never seen any person with the same set of values as another; they are completely unique to that individual. To ascertain values, I use a set of Personal Value Cards. On a large table, I set out five cards entitled: *Must Have, High Want, Want, Indifferent*, and *Don't Want* to function as column headings. The client holds the remaining seventy-five cards. Each one has a value written on it; the card could say, for example, *Freedom to Choose,* or *Honesty* or *Peace*.

The instructions to the client are: Think about a deep, rich, and satisfying life. In that life, where would each value belong? Must you have this value for your life to feel deep, rich, and satisfying? Would it be a *High Want*? Would it be a *Want*? Would you feel *Indifferent* about it? Would it be a *Don't Want*? Place the card in the column to which it belongs.

I sit and observe. In all cases, the client knows exactly where each value card belongs. When they have finished, I remove the cards they have placed under the headings *Want* and *Indifferent*, as they are not of high enough importance to discuss further. It *is* important for me to find out why the client has placed values in the *Must Have* and *High Want* categories. It is equally important to discuss the values placed in the *Don't Want* category, as it is not possible for someone to feel happy and fulfilled if a *Don't Want* value is having to be adhered to.

I then invite the client to define what each value means to them, as I know people will define each one in their own way. I also ask them to tell me why each value would be necessary for their life to feel deep, rich, and satisfying. In my experience, this is also easy for clients to verbalise. I think people do know at a visceral level what they want in their lives and they know how they have been designed; they simply have never been asked the questions that could effectively draw out such vital, but deeply buried information. At the end of our discussion, I read back notes I've taken as the client was speaking. This gives the person an overall report of what is required to have a life that feels rich, deep, and satisfying *for them.*

I ask the client to comment on any insights they gained about themselves while doing the exercise. I also ask permission to comment on what I have noticed while watching the person do the exercise. For example, I like to point out that I noticed how emphatically they placed a card such as *Freedom to Choose* under the *Must Have* column heading. This client has discovered that in order to live a full, rich, satisfying life, *Freedom to Choose* is essential! They experience a moment of insight when they realize that, until now, they have made most of their life choices according to what others wanted of them. It can be upsetting, however, if they realize they are at a point in their personal lives where they cannot really answer the question, what do I want to be *free to choose*? I reassure them that as we proceed in the life coaching process, this will become more and more apparent to them.

Not knowing what we want can adversely affect our dating life by keeping us from consciously choosing what we want in our intimate relationship. For instance, coaching clients have told me that they got married simply because everyone else around them was getting married. They had finished high school or university, and it was time to choose a mate and create a home and family. Clearly, choosing to marry because we know who we are and what we need and are now ready to co-create our lives, would be a more powerful perspective from which to make our choice of life partner.

If you would like to try doing the Personal Values exercise on your own at home, you can find the list of personal values that I use listed in Appendix 1.

What Do I Want? What I Want Points to What I Need

The American writer, Barbara Sher, published her book *Wishcraft* over three decades ago. Sher has been called the godmother of life coaching because she understood that to get what we want from life, we must first know *what* we want.

> There are plenty of hard-working, responsible men and women in our society who do know *how* to get things done but have never felt free to explore themselves and find out *what* they want to do... Contrary to what you may have been taught, there is nothing frivolous or superficial about what you want. It isn't a luxury that can wait until you've taken care of all the 'serious' business of life. It is a necessity. *What you want is what you need.* Your dearest wish comes straight from your core, loaded with vital information about who you are and who you can become. You've got to cherish it. You've got to respect it. Above all, you've got to *have* it. (xx-xxiii)

Sher's book is loaded with exercises to help us become clear about who we are, what we want, and how to get what we want. She makes the point that when we are very young we excel at knowing what we want and wishing for it. But somehow, many of us lose that ability. We may know what we hunger for, but somehow as we get older, we forget what it is. Perhaps as children we received messages that we must be content with what we had, because what we want seemed unrealistic to our parents; maybe we tried to reach some of our dreams and failed; maybe we were told by someone that we weren't smart enough or able enough, or maybe someone told us that *they* knew what we wanted, rather than allowing us to discover that for ourselves. Somebody said they knew what we wanted better than we did-- and we bought into it. For so many reasons, we may have adjusted our sights downward. We may have settled for what we thought we could reasonably attain, or we simply may have lost our ability to know what we truly want.

Today our work can become learning how to hunger, how to want, and how to dream again. We may even dare to dream for a wonderful, life-enhancing partner, and when we have done the necessary and exciting work of becoming a complete individual, we may even go about finding one. Without exception, life coaching clients of mine have experienced many moments of insight and clarity when they took the time to do the exercises in *Wishcraft*. I highly recommend them!

The Whole Life Grid: Intentionally Designing the Life I Want

I have found that teaching coaching clients about the concept of the Whole Life Grid helps them envision what it is to be a whole and complete person. This tool is described by Susan Jeffers in her book *Feel the Fear and Do it Anyway* (125-139).

Jeffers begins by showing us a picture called "Whole Life With Relationship," which is a box with the word Relationship written inside (128). Then she shows a picture entitled "Whole Life Without Relationship"; in this view the box is empty (128). This simple illustration helps us visualize why we can feel devastated by the loss of a significant person in our lives, especially a partner; we may realize that we made that person our "whole life." This happens when we invest so much of our time and emotional energy in the direction of one person that nothing else has any real significance to us. When that person dies, or chooses to end their relationship with us, we can feel completely bereft because we have identified our own Self so completely with that single individual. Realizing what we have done, we can consciously decide to make this loss an opportunity.

We can choose to grow and develop into a more mature adult for the sake of becoming even more healthy and whole. If we believe that a dynamic relationship is created by two whole people, then becoming a whole person becomes an exciting goal. Jeffers suggests we can create a more complete life patterned after the grid shape (129) as reproduced here. Creating a whole life grid can help us, in a very simple way, discover what elements constitute a life that feels complete, rich, and satisfying. How enlightening to realize that our entire life does not need to consist solely of the human being with whom we are in an intimate relationship. We can choose to make this relationship an important piece, but perhaps only a portion of our entire life! What freedom!

Contribution	Hobby	Leisure
Family	Alone Time	Personal Growth
Work	Relationship	Friends

We see that if our relationship with a significant other person is removed from the picture, we still have 8/9ths of a whole life remaining. Each day still holds the potential for experiences that bring us joy, fulfilment, and contentment. Thus, the loss of an intimate relationship in our life does not need to produce a feeling of emptiness and neediness. By designing our own personal whole life grid we can choose instead to live a life that reflects the diversity and the balance of Jeffer's helpful model. Creating a whole life grid creates the potential for a good day, each day.

Jeffers encourages us to "sculpt" our lives. She says most of us don't choose this option, but simply accept what comes to us and then complain about it. Rather than adopt this passive approach, Jeffers urges that we allow ourselves to know what we want, then go ahead and create what we need. For example, she suggests we think about who we want in our circle of friends, then take the initiative and make plans to get together. She advocates that we consider our bodies--what they would need to look and feel healthy--then go and do what is necessary (54).

Jeffers challenges us to realize that it is not another person's responsibility to make us happy. We get to be the one, and the *only* one, who can make ourselves happy! "What am I not doing in my life that I could be doing that I am blaming my partner for not doing for me?" (47) What a direct and helpful question! Jeffers confesses that when she took care of what needed to be handled in her own life, her anger toward others often dissolved. Of course, our intimate partners may be very caring and supportive of us. We can expect to have some needs met by our partner, for instance, our need to be supported in our personal growth, or, at times, our need to be nurtured. We need to know there is caring on our spouse's part, but "when we are not taking proper responsibility for our own lives, no amount of caring and nurturing suffices" (47).

The author James Hollis also addresses the folly of essentially handing over our lives to another human being. Hollis' account of our hunger for love is one we see represented in popular culture: we hope against hope for a *true love* to enter our lives;

we yearn for that special someone who will *complete us*, heal our lives and magically meet our deepest private need. We long for a love who will *be there* for us and generally make our lives right. Hollis calls this phantom figure "the magical other." He cautions that looking for such a person distracts us from realizing that these things are our own responsibility as we go through the process of our personal individuation (104).

This quest for a *rescuer-love* is not only a contemporary phenomenon. In 1844, the American journalist and women's rights advocate Margaret Fuller wrote her essay, "Women in the 19th Century." Fuller was a close friend of thinker and poet Ralph Waldo Emerson, and she was interested in world politics. But Fuller was equally devoted to her own education and personal growth, and cautioned those in her own century against what we in the twenty-first could term co-dependence. "If any individual live too much in relations, so that he becomes a stranger to the resources of his own nature, he falls after a while into a distraction, or imbecility, from which he can only be cured by a time of isolation, which gives the renovating fountains time to rise up" (qtd. in Thomas Moore, *Original Self* 135). Today, writer Thomas Moore credits Fuller for being "sharply aware of the tendency to find the soul's vitality exclusively in relationship with another, at the cost of one's own individuality" (134).

And so Hollis encourages each of us to develop our ability to be alone, lest we think that wholeness comes from fastening ourselves to someone else. "The capacity for solitude is a prerequisite for relationship with another. Otherwise it may well be that the desperate search for a partner is merely the expression of personal emptiness, and if that is the case, any relationship will be founded on weak grounds and will not satisfy the yearning for connection" (136). As Margaret Fuller put it so succinctly,

"Union is only possible to those who are units" (qtd. in Moore, 134).

Becoming a whole person is the developmental task of the second half of life, although if we are aware of the need to become a whole person--and what that means--it can become the developmental task we focus on at *any* time in our lives. I believe that in order to be the whole, healthy, happy, and free individual that we need to be in order to be a functional, happy person in a relationship, we need to know who we are and *be* who we are, taking full responsibility for our own happiness. If we form a relationship with another such individual, there is a far greater likelihood that we will be happy together.

Being a whole, healthy, happy, and free individual implies that we love ourselves and accept ourselves just as we are. For most of us, arriving at this place requires much personal growth and a lot of work. Healthy love-of-self is the key. Jesus instructed us to "love your neighbour *as yourself*" (*New International Version Bible*, Mark 12: 31). He makes it clear that we cannot love another unless we love ourselves. And he assumes that we *do* love ourselves. The ratio is exact: to the extent that we truly love and accept ourselves, that is the extent to which we can truly love and accept others. How, then, do we demonstrate our respect and love for others effectively? I look forward to sharing the tools for this divine task with you in Chapter Three, *We*!

I believe that the formula for personal wholeness consists of the following:

- knowing and living out our personality type,
- knowing our personal values and living highly in them,
- being aware that there is an original design for our lives, seeking it and living it out,
- awareness of the concept of the whole person grid and developing and living each area of our personal grid,
- being willing to take responsibility for our own personal fulfilment
- loving ourselves unconditionally.

It makes sense that if such individuals create a relationship with each other, they are bound to function well together! In the next chapter, I will discuss how we can more consciously choose the kind of partner who will be the best fit for us.

CHAPTER TWO

You:
How Do I Know You're the One for Me?

The consummation of our hopes in marriage happens not only through the daily testing of our ideals and our ability to bring those ideals alive in the partnership, but in the collision between the part of us that has great difficulty sustaining conversation with anything other than ourselves. Marriage is where we realize that the other person actually is alive and has notions and desires that have very little to do with our own hopes and dreams… Marriage is where we realize that we have married a stranger whom we must get to know… marriage is where all of these difficult revelations can consign us to imprisonment, or help us become larger, more generous, more amusing, more animated participants in the human drama.

David Whyte, *The Three Marriages: Reimagining Work, Self and Relationship*

Having spent a substantial amount of time thinking about how to become a whole and healthy human being, now it is time to consider our partner.

How do I get to know that "stranger" I am with?

Do I really know his or her hopes and dreams?

How can we, together, become "larger, more generous… animated participants" in the life we are sharing?

If we are not currently in a relationship, but looking to enter one, we must contemplate different but equally valuable questions.

Knowing who I am, what are my needs and wants in a relationship? Who would make a good match for me?

With whom can I create a healthy relationship and family?

What do I need to take into account so I choose a person who will be happy with me, too?

Asking ourselves practical questions like these are one of many things we can do to become more knowledgeable about people in general so that the person we marry will be less of a stranger to us. We can also access several tools to help us either choose a partner more consciously and wisely, or discover more about our current mate.

Relationship Values:
What I Want and Need in Intimate Relationship

When a client is seeking answers to some of the questions listed above, one of the first tools I use is a set of cards I developed called Relationship Value Cards. The cards are a deck of 70 words that denote characteristics most people consider when assessing a potential mate. (It's important to note that each individual will assign a different relative importance to each characteristic.) Examples of these values are: *Respect, Sexual Chemistry, Common Goals, and Loyalty.*

I ask my client to take each card and place it under one of the five heading cards included in the deck. Just as it is with the Personal Value Cards, the column headings are: *Must Have, High Want, Want, Indifferent, and Don't Want.* When my client has placed all the value cards, I ask him or her to look at each of the words that they have assigned to the *Must Have* and *High Want* categories.

Then I make a request of my client: Ask yourself what that word means to you, and why you value it so highly in a relationship.

It is equally important to consider the value cards that my client has assigned to the *Don't Want* category. These are characteristics that, if we identify them as present early in a new relationship, should make us want to run away, and run quickly! For example, if we have the value card that says *Wants Kids* in our *Don't Want* category and a new friend makes it clear that they want four children, pursuing the relationship only invites painful conflict.

Once we identify our *Must Have* and *High Want* values, we can develop a checklist to use early in new relationships. Sometimes it can be as simple as identifying that a person who doesn't love animals could never work out in the long run if we have designated *Loves Animals* as a *Must Have* value. Each individual must decide which Relationship Values are Must Haves for them. When we become clear about this, it allows us to find and enjoy relationships that are more fitting by avoiding predictable conflicts--conflicts that are *in the cards*.

I also use the Relationship Value Cards when someone is already in a serious relationship, but something doesn't feel quite right. The cards can quickly pinpoint what that "something" might be.

The cards can also be used to promote discussion within a couple. Each individual completes the relationship value assessment on their own, then, together with their partner, talks about what surprises them in their Relationship Values *Must Haves* and *Don't Wants*.

The Relationship Value Cards help us answer two questions: *who* do I want in an intimate relationship? and *what* do I want from my intimate relationship? I think the *who*, i.e. the character requirements we have, stay quite stable throughout our lifetimes, but the *what* we want can change.

When I discuss the *what* with young adults, they often wish to a join a good partner in buying a house, raising children, paying off student debts, saving for retirement, etc. When I talk about the *what* with people at midlife and beyond, often they are hoping for a companion with whom to enjoy leisure pursuits--someone who is willing and able to spend a lot of time with them, often simply sitting and talking and being together. At this time of life, a person of a more similar personality type is desirable, as it is easier to spend extended hours with someone who shares some of your interests and personality traits. In young adulthood, however, it seems beneficial to be with someone whose skills and interests are complementary. It makes sense that complementary skills in a couple might lead to the best chance of success in the tasks of raising a family and making the small business that is their marriage a success, too. This is one aspect of the reason couples who marry their opposite in the Myers Briggs personality typing system can do very well in young adulthood, but begin to struggle mightily after their children leave home.

The list of Relationship Values I use can be found in Appendix II at the back of the book. You can do the Relationship Value exercise for yourself and develop your own personalised list of *Must Have, High Wants,* and *Don't Want* Values.

The 4 "Cs": The Cornerstones of Relationship

After many conversations with people before, after, and during relationships that did *not* work out, I realized that consciously or unconsciously, we are all seeking 4 *"Cs"* that encompass in broader categories the individual values presented on the Relationship Value Cards.

The first *"C"* is *Character*. We look for a person of good character—a person of integrity. The book *Just Your Type*, by Tieger and Barron-Tieger, lists the aspects of relationship people find most important in a spouse. 95% of the people they surveyed said *Trust* was the most important element. This was closely followed by both *Communication* and *Mutual Respect* at 92%. 86% of respondents valued *Mutual Commitment* as the most important quality in their marriage. 82% said *Fidelity*. This research indicates that good Character is important to people of all personality types. "Even partners who are very different from each other can have a deep connection when they share these core values" (314).

The second *"C"* stands for *Chemistry*. We look for a person with whom we feel a strong sexual attraction. How and why we are attracted to another person is a mystery, but we know when we feel strongly attracted. They just *smell right* to us, and we know that our body loves being in their presence. Chemistry is one of the great mysteries and great joys of a relationship! There does not seem to be any direct correlation between personality type and chemistry, however, the way chemistry is experienced can vary. One NF/Intuitive Feeler life coaching colleague reported that when she was in a relationship with another NF/Intuitive Feeler, the sexual attraction felt like a soul-to-soul attraction, a soothing, calm warmth that filled her body. This same person reported that when she was in relationship with a person of an opposite personality type, she felt sexual attraction much more in her body than in her soul. She described it as being more of a "fiery, blood-boiling heat" or like being "branded by fire." She also remarked that popular movies tell us that the chemistry we feel with an opposite personality type is *real* love and the chemistry we feel with our soul mates is not truly love, but only friendship. She feels that both types of sexual attraction are equally valid and that we should not judge one type as better than the other.

The third *"C"* stands for *Common Values*. We seek a person who shares our values about such fundamental subjects as religion, children--or not, parenting, and lifestyle. For some people, having a partner who shares their religious beliefs is of paramount importance. Some people want material simplicity and would be miserable co-creating a life with a person who enjoys accumulating a lot of material goods. And for a union to be satisfying and harmonious, there has to be agreement about whether to have children, and if there will be children, how to raise them. These values need to be thoroughly explored before agreeing to commit to each other.

The fourth *"C"* stands for *Communication*. We look for a person with whom we can productively communicate about personal challenges as well as the challenges that will inevitably arise within the relationship. We seek someone with whom we can problem-solve. Communication is easier when a person shares our values, has good social skills, and is a person we respect and trust.

If we find a person who has the 4 *"Cs"* as we define them, then we have likely found a person with whom we can peacefully and happily co-exist. Now, there is one more *"C"* to consider.

The 5th C: What Is My Core Need?

Upon further conversation with coaching clients of many different personality types, I discovered that, for some of us, there is a *5th C*. I call it the *Core Need*. Especially for the NFs/Intuitive Feelers in the Myers Briggs personality system, there seems to be a certain something, in addition to the sensible 4Cs, that--if absent--will lead to a profound sense of dissatisfaction in a relationship, even if the all the other *"Cs"* are present. This Core Need can be difficult to name, because often the person is not aware of having it. They just know that something is missing in their intimate relationship.

I have found the best way to bring the Core Need to consciousness, and to name it, is to use the Relationship Value Cards. In the list of *Must Have* values something will show up, which upon discussion of its importance to the individual, produces a moment of profound insight. The person realizes that they have this need that they deeply want a partner to understand, and also meet, *even if it is an unspoken one*! Examples of Core Needs that I have seen in my work are "Gets Me," "Gives Me Space," or "Connection." This attribute or value is a soul need, and it is of utmost importance to get help to name it. As John O'Donohue said in his beautiful book, *Anam Cara*, "when you are understood, you are home. Understanding nourishes belonging. When you feel really understood, you feel free to release yourself into the trust and shelter of the other person's soul" (O'Donohue 14). For NFs in the Myers Briggs system, I have found that the meeting of this Core Need is the thing that produces the "in love" feeling that we crave. The feeling of physical attraction, induced by pheromones and sex hormones, is felt in the body, while the feeling of having the Core Need met is felt deep down in the soul.

In my experience, for most Sensors in the Myers Briggs system, the "in love" feeling does not require this 5th C. A Sensor seems to love in a different, less-complicated way than an Intuitive. They are looking for good communication, a character they can respect, common values, and physical chemistry. When these things are present, they can feel "in love." In my experience, the most satisfied marriages seem to occur between two Sensors because they usually don't require that hard-to-define 5th C, the *Core Need*. What they require is more easily measurable and therefore easier to meet. Of course, any pairing of any Myers Briggs personality typing can be satisfying, because when the 4Cs match up so much of what we require in marriage is satisfied. Yet, it cannot be denied that the NFs often seem to have that Core Need and they long to have it met in order to feel most contented in their relationships.

After all this consideration of what it means to love, and be "in love," I began to wonder if different personality types would define the meaning of the words *I love you* differently.

An ISFJ said, "I love you means I am committed to you to the end."
Another ISFJ said, "I love you means I feel safe and accepted and not judged by you."

An ENFP said, "I love you means I am here for you." Another ENFP said the exact same thing.

An ENFJ said, "I love you means I have a deep affection for you, including a sexual connection. You can count on me to always be your partner in life. I think you are wonderful and it makes me very happy to be with you."

An INFJ said, "I love you means I know in my heart that you are the one and that the search for the right fit for me is over. You "get" me, and I "get" you, so it feels wonderful to be partners.

We have the freedom to be authentic and transparent with each other. We cheer each other on, and we seek to understand each other, in total acceptance of what is, rather than what should be."

An INFP said, "I love you means my soul sees your soul and it is beautiful." Another INFP said, "I love you means I cannot believe the depth of my gratitude for you. I commit to being with you based on feelings of deep respect, admiration and a need for togetherness."

An ESTP said, "I love you means I admire you and I really enjoy sleeping with you."

An INTJ said, "I love you means you are loyal to me and you keep me safe."

An ISTJ said he notices that people say "I love you" when they seem to mean, "As long as you continue to make my life more pleasurable, you will continue to remain in my favour."

We can see that the simple words, *I love you*, mean different things to different people! We can't assume we know what those words mean until we become curious and ask our partners what they mean *for them*. I believe significant information about a person's Core Need can be found in what they mean when they say *I love you*. "*I love you,*" may be as much a statement about what the individual most deeply needs, as it is a statement about how they feel about their partner. Therefore, it is very helpful for each partner to consider what the words *I love you* mean to them and to share their definitions with each other. We all get to be who we are, and we all get to decide what *I love you* means to us, so no definition is either right or wrong. However, we gain valuable information from our partners by inquiring into this important question.

The 6th C: How Important Are Common Interests?

What fascinates me in our western culture of partnering up is that there does not seem to be a 6th C, *Common Interests*. One would think that a need to share common interests would be an important aspect of choosing a compatible intimate partner, but I have never seen a coaching client place Common Interests in his or her *Must Have* values. Could this be because I am almost always coaching people of opposite, or nearly opposite personality types? If so, it seems that people who choose to marry their opposite are using the 4*Cs* primarily to choose their partner. Could it be that this would be different if I were using the Relationship Value Cards and coaching people at midlife— people who are looking to marry a companion, rather than someone with whom to bear and raise children? Could it be that different phases of life, with their different tasks, lead us to choose different types of partners, and that we use different criteria at different times of the life cycle? This has been borne out in my experience. People looking to remarry in midlife seem more aware of having a Core Need, much more aware than they were in their twenties when choosing their first intimate partner.

I believe *Character, Chemistry, Common Values,* and *Communication* are always important, but at midlife the *Core Need*, especially for NFs, becomes critical to the decision-making process.

Myers Briggs Personality Type: The Importance of Personality Type in Intimate Relationship

Isabel Briggs Myers' original research showed that 35% of couples *not* in therapy had two of the four personality type letters in common; another 35% had three letters in common. Only 5% had no letters in common (*Gifts Differing: Understanding Personality Type,* 124). Briggs Myers said she was surprised by this, until she realized that most of her experience with married couples was with people she was, indeed, counselling. My own experience as a relationship coach bears this out, as 90% of the couples who see me for relationship coaching have no letters in common and the other 10% have only one letter in common!

In their book *Just Your Type,* Tieger and Barron-Tieger have compiled information specific to every possible personality type pairing. I make the couple aware of this, telling them that Tieger and Barron-Tieger have identified many of the joys of each personality pairing--*and* many of the frustrations. The authors also helpfully give us tips for each person in that pairing to interact more successfully with their partner. The couple read this information and then discuss it with each other, almost always creating moments of new insight. So many aspects--previously annoying and mysterious about each other and their relationship--suddenly make sense.

When we are married to a person of a very different personality type than our own, we can make a lot of faulty assumptions when that person does things that frustrate or annoy us. Sometimes we can even feel pity for other people not being able to think like we do! We can feel that the person is trying to annoy us on purpose, or they are not normal, or something is desperately wrong with them, when actually, they are simply being who they are.

We discover that, just as form follows function, behaviour follows personality type. Not taking the behaviour of a person of a different personality personally is the beginning of making the relationship more functional. Not making the assumption that behaviour you don't agree with or understand is meant to annoy you, is another step toward an even better relationship. Developing an *attitude of curiosity* is instantly helpful because curiosity is not accompanied by judgement. When people treat each other with criticism or contempt, a relationship cannot thrive; a strong possibility exists that it will break down for that reason alone. But when two people approach each other like scientists who are seeking to understand each other, a good, functional relationship becomes possible.

In their research, Tieger and Barron-Tieger found that about 10% of couples share all four personality type letters, about 20% share three letters, roughly 35% have only two letters in common, approximately 25% have one letter in common and 10% have no letters in common (*Just Your Type,* 313). They found that the more similar individuals are to their partners, the more satisfied they are with their relationships (313).

It makes sense that the more Myers Briggs personality type letters people have in common, the easier it may be for them to communicate effectively. In fact, Tieger and Barron-Tieger's research confirms that the more type preferences a couple have in common, the higher they rated the quality of their communication. Also, respondents in their survey report effective communication as second only to trust as the most important component of a satisfying relationship. 92% of respondents considered good communication "the most important" aspect of a satisfying relationship. The more satisfied they are with the quality of their communication, the more satisfied they are with their relationship (313). I have come to realize that we can assume everyone else is just like us, and if they are not, we can think that they are not *normal*; sometimes we can even see others as *weird* or *broken* if they are very different from us.

Of course, the truth is that each of the 16 distinct personality types is normal and each one has equal worth and value. We all have the right to be and to know who we are born to be. Our personality type is not a choice; it is an orientation. I have come to see that very subtly, we can still expect people to be just like us, that our way is the right way. It remains difficult to really realize *and accept* that there are 16 distinct personality types, all of which have an equal right to exist, to be respected, and to live in peace in this world. A very high level of understanding, wisdom, and empathy seems to be required to truly understand and live this knowledge in our day-to-day lives. This harkens back to David Whyte's passage at the beginning of this chapter. "The other person actually has notions and desires that have very little to do with our own... Marriage is where we realize that we have married a stranger who we must get to know" (263).

For example, I was doing the Personal Values assessment with a woman who is ESFJ/Extroverted, Sensing, Feeling, Judging and to my surprise, she placed the value, *Transparency*, in the *Don't Want* category. Intrigued, I asked her to explain. She said, "I don't want to come into a room and have people not see that I am there. I don't want them to look right through me! I want to make an impact when I come into a room. I don't want to ever be ignored."

When doing the values assessment with a person who is INFP/Introverted, Intuitive, Feeling, Perceiving, I saw the value *Transparency* defined very differently. This individual placed the card in the opposite category, as a *Must Have*. This INFP told me that, for him, *Transparency* is the most important value. His highest dream and goal is to be able to look into someone's soul and to have them be able to look into his. This difference in defining the value card *Transparency* illustrates how dangerous and misleading it can be for me to assume that my definition of any value is either correct or the only one. We need others to complete our awareness. We need to be open to realizing that others think differently than we do, and in being open to others' ideas and perceptions, we can grow as unique individuals.

Explaining the difference in the way people see such core concepts as personal values can also provide moments of insight when we begin to realize how different people's perspectives can be based on the orientation of their personality type. And that no one is ever wrong just because they see things differently!

Openness to other ways of being and seeing the world is essential to extending unconditional love, acceptance, and support to our intimate partners. When we withhold unconditional love and acceptance from those closest to us, we begin to judge them and find them wrong, simply for being who they are. This creates emotional strain and stress in the relationship. If, instead, we find joy in the difference, we create the possibility for mutual respect and enjoyment of each other.

Now that we have explored Me and You, it is time to consider the relationship that we will create. What are some of the tools we need to create the healthiest possible relationship for us? This is what we will explore in our next chapter, named with a wink and a nod to artistic license. Welcome to *We*!

CHAPTER THREE   We:
                    Learning to Become a Couple

After two individuals fall in love and the heady first days of love are behind them, each person begins a discernment process regarding whether they wish to proceed toward becoming a couple, either for now or forever. Each must think about what they really value in a relationship--what their top relationship values are and how closely their new beloved matches those *Must Have* criteria. Each person must consider both *who* do I want and need in an intimate relationship and *what* do I want and need in an intimate relationship. The more consciously aware they become of their unique requirements, the more likely they are to be able to discover whether this partner is a good choice for them.

If the prospective partner seems to be a "fit," these two individuals will become a couple. Until this point, the relationship has looked like two people enthralled with each other and then two people checking each other out. Now, they each begin to discover if they can create their unique *"We"* in peace, contentment, and mutual agreement.

Just as brand-new parents have been known to jump into the car on their first Friday home and go out for pizza--then remember there is a baby in the crib upstairs, so, too, can each partner in a new relationship sometimes continue to operate autonomously, forgetting there is a new *We* that is very real and requires every bit as much care as a new baby in the home of a young couple.

Learning to operate as *We* can be awkward! Learning how to converse respectfully as *We*, sharing feelings and thoughts with each other, is very different from two people taking turns *telling* the other something. When the skill of sharing is present, the conversation flows; it operates like gears meshing on a bike, rather than grinding with fits and starts. For instance, one person may have a slower pace of thinking and sharing than the other. Since it is not advisable for a person to operate at anything other than their natural pace, the higher-ramped individual could learn to slow down internally and share at their partner's pace for the sake of their developing *We*. The new couple has to learn what the tempo of sharing looks like for them, together. This takes commitment, consciousness, a sense of humour, and patience to achieve! It is not unlike learning to play a new instrument. And like discovering any new skill, we must acknowledge that learning the art of conversation with our beloved does not necessarily come naturally--as is portrayed in movies--but takes intention, attention, and time given to practise. And just as when we learn to play an instrument, mastering the art of communicating with our partner is worth the effort.

Learning to operate as a *We*, developing a two-as-one consciousness, is like learning to run a three-legged race. First we submit to having our ankles tied to our partner's. Then we put our arms around each other, agreeing to run the race together. (This part feels great!) And then, we try to move forward…. Initially, this part feels awkward! We are moving from the idea of being a couple, which we love, into the practice of becoming a couple, which is hard work. We are moving from the dreaming place into the everyday, consensus reality level of putting our dreams into practice, from intention to manifestation.

Just as when we practise for the three-legged race, this putting into practise--this manifestation stage--requires much co-operation and conversation as the couple finds their own unique way to move forward. They will try, and fail. After failing, they will recover. And they will go through the cycle of practise/fail/

recover many times. What fuels the willingness to continue to practise? Love!

It helps to know that two people committed to moving from functioning as two autonomous individuals to functioning as a couple is not a given and is not easy. They may have made the assumption that *if we really love each other*, it should feel effortless to mesh and become a couple. This is a fallacy. The idea that we love each other and the idea that we want to come together as a couple are separate concepts. We can be guilty of collapsing these two concepts into one, thus producing the above assumption that all will be wine and roses. If we separate the two ideas and think about them consciously, they could look more like: one, we love each other, and two, we commit, therefore, to learning how to become, and operate well, as a couple.

When we are conscious and present, open and flexible with each other, being willing to bend and flow with our process of adjustment, we stand the best chance of learning how to become a healthy *We* who can enjoy being *We* as much as we enjoy being Me. Of course, just as there are times when we don't like the challenges of being an autonomous single person, there will be times when we feel frustrated by being a yoked-together couple, struggling and resisting each other. The key to dealing with these occasions is to be honest and transparent with our partner, trying to be aware within ourselves how we are feeling and then sharing that respectfully with hope and trust in our partner. And with hope and trust in our relationship. Even with this knowledge, we will have to practise, fail, and recover, but it seems that with each cycle, trust grows--and with it--the commitment and facility to run the three-legged race together.

The Five Love Languages of Relationship: Five Key Ways We Give and Receive Love

In service of helping a couple develop their sense of being a *We*, I have found that one of the most eye-opening, effective, efficient tools I can teach them is something called the Five Love Languages.

Dr. Gary Chapman wrote a book by this name in 1992. He teaches us that each human being has an "emotional love tank" that is filled in five different ways (23). The Five Love Languages include:

1. Words of Affirmation: offering verbal compliments or words of appreciation or praise that build up or encourage another person

2. Quality Time: giving your undivided attention by listening intently, participating with a person in an activity that has meaning for them, or looking at each other and talking

3. Giving Gifts: thinking of your loved one and taking the time and trouble to acquire a thoughtful gift

4. Acts of Service: doing things for your loved one that you know they would like you to do, seeking to please your loved one by helping them or serving them

5. Physical Touch: hugging, kissing, holding hands and/or having sexual intercourse is a powerful vehicle for some individuals to communicate emotional intimacy and experience love

After explaining each love language, I ask each partner which of these languages makes them feel most loved. Their answer reveals their primary love language. We tend to try to express love to others in our own language. If our partner's love language is different from ours, speaking in our primary love language will not be as successful, of course, as if we speak in theirs. For example, if my own primary love language were words of affirmation, I would try to show my love and appreciation by praising my partner's efforts at maintaining our yard. However, if my partner's primary love language were giving gifts, I would better succeed in showing my love and appreciation by giving my partner a new t-shirt or mower attachment. Similarly, while it would be natural for my generous spouse to buy me a new bike, what I would *really* like is to hear him say how much he enjoys biking with me. These words of affirmation (my primary love language) would make me feel loved and cared for. It is rare for a couple in counselling to share the same love language. In fact, it's often the case that the least natural way for one partner to show love is the very behaviour that is the primary love language for their mate. Learning to speak your partner's primary love language takes discipline, similar to learning to speak a foreign language, but the payoff can be immense. According to Chapman, a full emotional love tank is the key to making a marriage work. Just as in trying to acquire any new habit, practise makes perfect. You can go to www.5lovelanguages.com to take the test for yourself!

Don't Take Anything Personally; Instead, Choose To Be Curious:
A Precept for Attaining Personal Peace in Relationship

When we learn how to not take anything anyone says personally, it is nothing short of life-transforming because inwardly, we become free. And when we feel free, we are in the best possible place to put our full attention on our beloved and to be as conscious as possible about our budding *We*. What does it mean not to take anything personally and how do we put it into practise?

Don Miguel Ruiz defines this concept in his very useful book, *The Four Agreements.*

> Nothing other people do is because of you. It is because of themselves. All people live in their own dream, in their own mind; they are in a completely different world from the one we live in. When we take something personally, we make the assumption that they know what is in our world, and we try to impose our world on their world.
>
> Even when a situation seems so personal, even if others insult you directly, it has nothing to do with you. What they say, what they do, and the opinions they give are according to the agreements they have in their own minds. Their point of view comes from all the programming they received during domestication...
>
> When you take things personally, then you feel offended, and your reaction is to defend your beliefs and create conflicts. You make something big out of something so little, because you have the need to be right and make everyone else wrong. You also try hard to be right by giving your own opinions. In the same way, whatever you feel and do is just a projection of your own personal dream, a reflection of your own agreements. What you say, what you do, and the opinions you have are according to the agreements you have made and these opinions have nothing to do with me. (48-50)

As we consider our relationships, we do well to ponder Ruiz's words. I think we *do* tend to take things personally, especially when we love and feel attached to the person speaking. Because we love them, their opinion of us matters greatly and because we are attached to them, we fear losing them. When we become aware of this, we can choose another way. We can choose to come from the perspective of curiosity with our loved ones, rather than the *I'm right and you're wrong* or the *I'm afraid of losing you* perspective. When we listen to our loved one from a perspective of openness and curiosity--without a need to be right, without a need to impress our viewpoint upon them and with a willingness to listen with an open heart to their heart--conflict in our relationship diminishes dramatically. In addition, once we realize that we should take nothing personally, we realize that if a person is coming at us with a lot of hurtful talk, it reflects their own feelings of being hurt and in pain. Then, from the perspective of curiosity, we can choose to ask ourselves why they might be feeling hurt and upset and approach them with compassion and empathy. This is what it means not to take something personally.

Likewise, if a person tells us we are wonderful, we can realize it is likely that person is feeling wonderful themselves right now. Strangely enough, though we enjoy being told we are wonderful, it may be wise to receive these words with the understanding that the compliment is coming our way from the inner place of our beloved feeling very positive about themselves at that particular time. We can choose not to be too affected by anything anyone says, whether we are told we are wonderful, or we are told we are the worst person who ever walked the face of the earth. Actually, we are being subjected to that person's range of emotions, the range of experience within their internal world. As Ruiz says, "You eat all their garbage, and now it becomes your garbage. But if you do not take it personally, you are immune in the middle of hell" (49).

Rather than choosing to take things personally, we can attain more emotional freedom and peace in our relationships by choosing to adopt the useful perspective of curiosity. From this powerful place, we are able to feel strong and act strong in service of building the most whole and healthy *We* that we can possibly create.

The Three Levels of Reality: For Happiness in Intimate Relationship, We Must Be Aware of Each of Them

In his book, *Dreaming While Awake: Techniques for 24-Hour Lucid Dreaming,* eminent Jungian psychoanalyst and physicist, Arnold Mindell teaches us that there are three levels of reality. These are called The Dreaming, Dreamland, and Consensus Reality (15). Our intimate relationships operate on all three levels. For instance, when we first catch a glimpse of someone across a room and sense there is a possibility for a relationship with that person, we are in the Dreaming level of the relationship. It is a wordless place, full of possibility. When we walk across the room and begin to converse with this new person, we enter the Dreamland phase of relationship. We know nothing about the individual, but we eagerly begin to discover things about them and then start dreaming about what could possibly happen in our liaison with them.

Later on, if we decide to form a relationship and spend enough time with this person, we enter the Consensus Reality phase of the relationship. This is the concrete everyday level of relating. For instance, a couple who may have been attracted across the room (The Dreaming level), then struck up a conversation and began to date (Dreamland level), will--should they establish a partnership—eventually have to decide who does the dishes and who takes out the garbage (Consensus Reality level). This level is very practical and at the same time, not very romantic!

All relationships tend to proceed toward Consensus Reality, but an intimate relationship requires healthy doses of the Dreaming and Dreamland level experiences to survive and thrive. This is why we need to celebrate birthdays and anniversaries, spend time sitting on the couch talking face-to-face and holding hands, and go out on regular date nights. These experiences give the dreaming level of experience a chance to live on. The Dreaming and Dreamland levels are where the magic and fun and joy of relationship live.

I teach couples about the three levels of reality and encourage them to remain conscious of the need to keep The Dreaming and Dreamland levels of the relationship alive and well. I also encourage them to use their imaginations in this pursuit.

The Five Love Languages, Don't Take Anything Personally; Instead Choose to be Curious, and The Three Levels of Reality are three skills I teach couples in service of building their relationship. There are two more concepts I use with almost all couples who come to see me when they are struggling in their relationship. Both concepts help the couple gain a bigger picture of their situation and give them effective tools to do something about it.

The Four Horsemen of Relationship: Four Relationship Killers

*John Gottman wrote a wonderful book called The Seven
Principles for Making Marriage Work.* In it, he draws upon the
four horsemen of the Apocalypse. In their original Biblical form,
the four horsemen are harbingers of the Last Judgment, bringing
upon the world conquest, war, famine, and death. In his book,
Gottman applies the symbolic horsemen to four specific, negative
behaviors that may exist in a marriage, behaviours "which if
allowed to run rampant, are lethal to a relationship" (27).

The first Horseman is *Criticism.* Gottman explains that we all
have complaints about our intimate partners, but there is a big
difference between a complaint and a criticism. A complaint
addresses what our partner *does*; a criticism speaks negatively
about who our partner *is.* For example, we can say, "I'm
disappointed that you didn't do the laundry last night, like you
said you would, and now I haven't got a clean shirt to wear to
work today." This is a valid complaint. If we said, "You don't
care about me. You only think of yourself. You said you would
do the laundry and you didn't. Now I don't have a clean shirt to
wear to work today." This is criticism, as we have linked doing or
not doing the laundry with the character and intentions of our
partner and made the assumption that not doing the laundry was
intended to hurt us. We can work with complaints objectively,
but criticism damages our relationship.

The second Horseman is *Contempt.* Contempt doesn't stop at
criticism; it amps it up and adds sarcasm, belittling, cynicism,
name-calling, and hostile humour to interactions.

In whatever form, contempt--the worst of the four
horsemen--is poisonous to a relationship because it
conveys disgust. It is virtually impossible to resolve a
problem with your partner when your partner is getting

the message you're disgusted with him or her.
Inevitably, contempt leads to more conflict rather than
to reconciliation. (29)

The third Horseman is *Defensiveness.* Although it's
understandable that we will try to defend ourselves when we are
in conflict with our partner, research shows this approach rarely
has the desired effect because the attacking spouse experiences
their partner's defensiveness as a way of blaming him or her.
When we defend ourselves we are saying, in effect, "The
problem isn't *me,* it's *you"* (31). Gottman asserts that
defensiveness--rather than leading to empathy and compassion--
tends to escalate conflict and this is what makes it so deadly.

The fourth Horseman is *Stonewalling.* This includes cutting off
communication, the silent treatment, refusal to engage, and
withdrawal. Gottman says this is usually the last Horseman to
appear in a relationship because "it takes time for the negativity
created by the first three Horsemen to become overwhelming
enough for stonewalling to become an understandable 'out'"
(34).

When I work with couples, I am reminded to introduce them to
the Four Horsemen whenever I see one or both parties using one
of these tactics. I've discovered that couples who use the four
horsemen as a matter of course are usually unaware they are
doing so. And they are grateful to be taught alternative strategies.
In Gottman's book he explains how to deal with each of the Four
Horsemen when they appear--both to increase the skill level of
the couple and to make them conscious of how harmful they can
be to their relationship.

*Fail and Recover: We Will Fail in Our Intimate Relationships;
It's How We Handle It That Matters*

One of the keys to making a relationship work is to be aware that
we *will* fail our partners *and* that this is not the end of the world.
Rather than an opportunity to throw in the towel, this malfunction
can be an opportunity to practise the strategy called Fail and
Recover. In 2009, I participated in a nine-month-long leadership
program offered by Coaches Training Institute. One of the most
important characteristics, we were told, of a mature leader is not
that they never fail, but that when they do fail, they are willing to
know their impact, take responsibility for their impact, and stay
around to clean up their impact. Mature people accept they will
fail and they commit themselves to recover when they do.

Likewise in our intimate relationships, despite our best intentions
to always be good and kind to our spouses, there will be times
when we fall short. Accepting that we are human and that we *will*
fail makes it easier to acknowledge our failures, take
responsibility for our impact, ask forgiveness, then pick up the
pieces and carry on.

A friend once told me that he believes the oft-quoted line from
Erich Segal's 1970 romance, *Love Story,* in which the hero
proclaims, *Love means never having to say you're sorry.*
Personally, I think nothing could be further from the truth! For
me, love means never wanting to cause your partner pain—and
when you do—wanting to say, "I am sorry I hurt you and I hope
to never do that again, dear." Failing or hurting our intimate
partner is not the biggest sin, not at all. Not caring enough to
sincerely apologise is a much bigger failing. In fact, we can come
to the place where we are so humble within ourselves and within
our relationship, that apologising comes easily, and failing, and
then recovering, becomes something both partners learn to excel
at.

I have found a simple technique called "Making I Statements" so helpful here. When I feel wounded, it is better to say, "That hurt!" or "I feel hurt," rather than to say, "*You* make me mad!" Making my complaint, or stating my emotional pain starting with "I feel..." is much less likely to provoke a defensive response and much more likely to cause my partner to go toward a perspective of curiosity.

Of course, we strive to do better in our interactions. Both partners in a relationship intend to love and serve each other with excellence and compassion. But we are both so darn human that something like a frustrating day at work can make our best intentions seem impossible to fulfil. As human beings we can be deeply self-centered. We seem to put our own best interests first, despite our wish to do otherwise. However, having accepted that we will fail--and then learning how to recover quickly *and well*-- is a relationship skill worth its weight in gold.

When we own our faults and failings, there is something disarming about being vulnerable, authentic, open, and transparent; it seems to have the power to melt the hardest human heart. We become mirrors of each other's humanity. There is something about being the opposite of self-protective, rationalizing, blaming, and defensive that is appealing and healing. It is worth the risk we take that if we open ourselves to our spouse, they may hurt us back, be critical or contemptuous of us, or stonewall. If they do react in these ways to a sincere apology, then their response is not about us; it is about them and where they are in their lives. We must not take it personally.

Let us dare to learn how to fail and recover, learn how to apologise and accept with humility that we will need to be forgiven at times. This is good for our mental, emotional, physical, and spiritual health. As I write, I am reminded of the famous chapter in the Bible and these timeless, wise, and beautiful words.

> If I speak in the tongues of men and of angels, but have not love, I am only a resounding gong, or a clanging cymbal. If I have the gift of prophecy and can fathom all mysteries and all knowledge, and if I have a faith that can move mountains, but have not love, I am nothing. If I give all I have to the poor and surrender my body to the flames, but have not love, I gain nothing.
>
> Love is patient, love is kind. It does not envy, it does not boast. It is not proud. It is not rude. It is not self-seeking, it is not easily angered. It keeps no record of wrongs. Love does not delight in evil, but rejoices with the truth. It always protects, always trusts, always hopes, always perseveres.
>
> Love never fails.
>
> (*New International Version*, 1 Corinthians. 13.1-8)

When we fail to show our love, there is only one thing to do. Be aware of our impact on our partner. We have hurt them! We need to allow ourselves to feel what we have done. Then we need to apologise, promptly and sincerely. And accept the words that our spouse may need to speak to us about our impact. Then decide together to forgive, forget, and carry on. Intimate partners who learn and practise this skill will reap the benefits.

Learning how to fail and recover gracefully may be one of the most important skills of intimate relationship. This is how our *We* can become characterised by competent compassion. In the meantime, we fall... we scrape our knees, we clean them, we bandage them and we move forth together into the world, maybe limping a bit, but always hand-in-hand, living in hope and developing in grace. Learning how to fail and recover serves the development of our relationship just as it is a profound part of the process of learning to become whole individuals, because learning to fail and recover helps us, as human beings, to grow in empathy, compassion, humility, and selflessness.

We have learned a lot about *Me, You and We*--about who we need to be in order to engage in a healthy relationship, about who and what we need in our intimate partner, and how to interact well once we have found each other. Now it is time to return to the woman in our opening story, a woman who was married to her partner of many years and suffering from the pain, loneliness, and confusion of not knowing what was going wrong for her in her life and in her relationship. Let us look more deeply now into the problem of Soul Misery in Relationship; if we are suffering from it, what can we do about it? This is what we will discuss next in the chapter, *Love the Question.*

CHAPTER FOUR   Love the Question:
                 What Is Going On in Midlife Relationships?

In my experience as a life coach serving many couples who are
struggling, I believe that what precipitates Soul Misery in
Relationship is being with a partner who is close to being one's
exact opposite, according to Myers Briggs typology. Often, this
person is, indeed, our opposite. For reasons we have discussed,
building a life with our opposite may serve us well during the
childrearing phase, but once we enter midlife, suddenly, living
with our opposite can feel jarring, unsettling, and unfulfilling in
ways we do not initially understand. When we are young adults,
being with someone whose nature is quite different from our own
provides us with a partner whose skills complement our own.
Together, we add up to a powerful combination of all the skills
we need to succeed at creating a functional relationship for
establishing a home and competently raising our children. When
we reach midlife and our children begin to grow independent, we
can find ourselves wanting a different kind of mate--someone
who shares our interests, someone who loves to talk with us,
someone who is more of a companion to enjoy life--someone
whose personality type is very similar to ours. This shift in our
needs can happen subtly and gradually over time, sometimes so
subtly that apparently out-of-the-blue, one day our partner can
feel all wrong for us. Being with someone who once seemed
entirely satisfactory, then suddenly seems unsuitable, can be very
disconcerting and upsetting.

Not only can what we want in a partner change when we reach
middle age, this is a time in life when we begin to ask questions
of ourselves: *who am I* and *why am I here?* We may experience a
drive to become *all* that we are born to be. As James Hollis
teaches us, we yearn to "individuate," as discussed in Chapter

One. If early adulthood is usually spent focussing on the needs of others, now we feel a pull to direct our energies toward reaching our personal potential.

One soul misery sufferer described her experience as disappearing into a void. *"Soul Misery in Relationship felt like a dark, bottomless hole that I very slowly found myself sinking deeper and deeper into. It was insidious; little by little I became more and more lost without knowing why. Nothing in my life had changed--same wonderful man, same children, same job that I loved, same life in general. It was devastating to imagine that the love of my life and father of my children for more than twenty years was the least likely person in the world who could understand me or help me find my way back to peace and contentment. The more energy I invested into saving our relationship, the deeper into the vortex I fell. I had to make an impossible choice: save myself or save my relationship."*

Author Brené Brown calls this time of life the *midlife unravelling.* You feel a desperate pull to live the life you 'want' to live, not the one you're 'supposed' to live. The unravelling is a time when you are challenged by the universe to let go of who you think you are supposed to be and to embrace who you are. (Brown xiii)

We are pulled inexorably to do this work. It takes a lot of time. A lot of questions arise. And we must learn to love the questions and develop an ability to co-exist with the questions for a lengthy period of time. This work is slow, sometimes laborious and requires much processing and integration of what we discover along the way.

Each Soul Misery in Relationship sufferer is living within their own unique relationship. It is a one-of-a-kind situation. There is no one-size-fits-all solution. Thus, the best advice I can give

somcone in this situation is not to rush the process of unra\
or of remaking yourself. It is like the process of metamorph
In the cocoon, a caterpillar's body is broken down into som\
called imaginal cells. These cells are undifferentiated and, like
stem cells, can become any type of cell. The caterpillar is remade
into a new creation, a beautiful butterfly. Likewise, if we are
willing to submit to the whole process of metamorphosis, we will
emerge beautiful and whole and free. We must resist cutting into
the cocoon of our transformation too soon. With butterflies, if
you cut into their cocoon before the metamorphosis process is
complete, the butterfly dies. Likewise with us. If we rush the
process in our haste to escape the pain of unravelling or the work
of transformation, something essential is always lost.

Watching a video of metamorphosis, I was struck by how long it
takes the caterpillar to let go of the branch and drop into the
chrysalis. (www.vimeo.com/7203408) We can know that we
need to, and want to, enter the midlife unravelling process, yet it
can be so difficult to let go of life as we know it and begin the
metamorphosis. We cannot be assured of the end result. And it
can be challenging to enter willingly into the unknown.

Swiss psychologist, Carl Jung, was known to say, *What you resist
persists*. If we refuse to submit to the process of personal growth
when we need to do it, the result is a colourless and unhappy life.
Sometimes ill health can result. We may try to assuage our
emotional numbness with alcohol, food, or other drugs. It can be
difficult to prioritise our own personal growth when there are so
many competing demands on our time: our families, our careers,
our friendships, our community service--yet, we must be aware
that if we do not choose to grow and develop we will suffer
personal consequences such as physical illness or emotional
"grayness."

I have sat alongside many individuals suffering from Soul Misery in Relationship as they went through their period of transformation. The process occurs in steps and stages. We can feel that we have completed our personal metamorphosis and feel so relieved about it, but so often another stage of growth will reveal itself and we need to enter another cycle of change. In fact, I think it is likely that for most of us, individuation can take a lifetime. Thus, it becomes important that we begin to love our questions and be willing to submit to the process of life, rather than demand a certain end result at any given time. We can even begin to develop a taste for taking the next step and enjoy a sense of anticipation about it! Sometimes our next step is not clear at all, and we must sit patiently waiting for it to be revealed. But once it is revealed, it feels wonderful when we learn to submit to the process, trusting that the next step, and the next, will be revealed to us when the time is right. Just as the "solution" or resolution of personal Soul Misery is unique to the individual, so the "solution" to Soul Misery in Relationship is always unique to the relationship, as unique as each of the individuals in the relationship and as unique as the relationship itself.

Our highest goal, overall, is to attain deep personal congruence. Deep personal congruence occurs when we are living in line with our values and inhabiting a powerful perspective about our lives and our relationships. We are not having pesky persistent physical symptoms that point us to realize there is something we are not conscious of, something we are afraid of seeing and dealing with. When we are in deep personal congruence, we feel content, fulfilled, and deeply satisfied within the core of ourselves, and although we can be affected by the external circumstances of our lives, within ourselves, we feel settled and at peace.

When I work with couples at midlife, I almost always work with them individually, seeing one partner one week and the other partner the next. I do so because each partner has their own individuation process to complete and this takes precedence over their relationship work. I encourage each of them to become as "whole" and "complete" as possible before we look at their relationship. In most instances, once each partner has done their own work, they turn to each other and find that their relationship is workable, whereas before their metamorphosis work, they were feeling irritated and upset with their mate. They may need to become aware of, and learn how to use, some of the tools in the relationship toolkit, but most often, because they are both people of good Character, sharing Common Values, good Communication, and good physical Chemistry, they find they have enough in common to continue on in their relationship.

However, sometimes this does not turn out to be the case. Sometimes there are too many factors that add up to an unworkable situation for one or both of the partners. For instance, the couple may find they no longer have any Common Interests; they can't meet each others' Core Need; they can't Communicate in such a way as to feel emotionally connected. They may have talked about the situation together for hours, read countless self-help books, given time for things to change, and sought counselling. And yet, they still cannot seem to find a way to make the relationship feel sustainable and nourishing for both of them. What should they do then? We will discuss this situation in our next chapter, *Breaking Up Is Hard to Do*.

CHAPTER FIVE   Breaking Up Is Hard to Do:
What If You Want to End the Relationship?

You may have read this book thus far and come to the conclusion that yours is a marriage of opposite--or near opposite--personality types. You may have become aware of who you are, and now understand that there is no "magical other," that you are responsible for your own individuation. You may have become aware of who your partner is, too. You may realize that in this partner you have the *4Cs*: good *Communication* regarding your home and children; good *Chemistry*; shared *Common Values*; and your spouse may well be a person of good *Character*. And yet, you have come to see that you have a *Core Need* that is not being attended to--and you may feel desperate to have that Core Need met. For instance, you may crave intellectually stimulating conversation. Or, you may need meaningful emotional connection; you may desire that your personal vision of life be understood by your partner in a real and profound way. You may need to feel cherished. Perhaps you need a lot of physical touch and have not been receiving it. You may have been married for a long time--so long that you and your family are part of established communities, communities that you have no wish to disrupt.

And yet, you are aware of a gray feeling in your soul, a feeling of despair, especially when you are alone with your good spouse for lengthy periods of time, not distracted by tasks that need doing or the people you normally relate to. It is exceedingly painful to realize that such a good person is no longer a person with whom you want to spend much time. For instance, you may find the idea of a vacation, just the two you, unappealing.

As difficult as it is, it is time to face the fact that you are not happy in your relationship and it is time to allow yourself to think deeply about whether you want to stay. Allowing oneself to consider leaving one's marriage is terrifying for most of us. You wonder what people will think. Will they treat you the same, or will they judge you if you choose to leave your "good" marriage to a "good" person? And you wonder if they will criticize you if you choose to leave for "no good reason."

How do we allow our minds to even begin to approach this frightening topic? I think it helps to step back and try to see the bigger picture of the intimate relationship in general, the bird's-eye view perspective.

In her book *Coming Apart,* author Daphne Kingma confirms that intimate relationships provide us with "emotional communion, circumstantial companionship, an environment for childrearing and an economic backup" (135). She also says that an intimate partnership can help us meet goals we have set for ourselves. And so, on an unconscious level, "when we establish a relationship, we are not just 'falling in love,' we are choosing the person and kind of relationship that will help us accomplish our developmental task of the moment" (135).

Knowing that we choose a partner--even if it has been an unconscious choice--in order to accomplish a developmental task can help us not judge ourselves so harshly as we consider ending our relationship. Perhaps we are not stupid, a failure, a person of bad judgment or of reprehensible character. It may simply be that our current developmental task has been completed and we do not view our current partner as the one to accompany us into our next developmental task.

For instance, we may marry the first time hoping to achieve the developmental task of co-creating a family: buying a home, and conceiving, birthing, and raising children. When those tasks are done, we can then move on at midlife to the task author James Hollis says we must accomplish, the task of individuation--knowing who we are and becoming all we are meant to be (*Finding Meaning in the Second Half of Life*, 10). It takes other human beings to complete our awareness of ourselves. Ideally, we want a partner who can understand what it means for our personality type to individuate, and we want that partner to be interested, willing, and able to help us navigate our individuation process. In short, it makes sense to be in an intimate relationship with someone who is of similar personality type to us during this time. Tieger and Barron-Tieger's research (which we discuss in Chapter Two) bears this out. I believe at this time of life, a Sensor naturally does better with a Sensor, and an Intuitive naturally does better with an Intuitive. Why would this be so?

In the bestselling book about the Myers Briggs personality typing system, *Gifts Differing,* Isabel Briggs Myers discusses the difference between the preference of sensing (S) and the preference of intuition (N). Sensors take in, depend on, and trust information that comes from their five senses. Information that comes from other people in the form of words is less trustworthy to them in and of itself. In order for language to mean something, words have to be translated into real-life experience. In contrast to this way of receiving information, Intuitives are not interested in--and are often bored by--reports of things the way they are. Intuitives are excited by--and interested in--the information that comes from their unconscious. These intuitions, or hunches, lead them to think about possibilities for the future: ideas to explore; conversations to have; books to be written. The Intuitive personality trusts what they know by way of the intuitions they experience (Gifts Differing, 57, 58). Thus, conversations between a Sensor and an Intuitive can be very frustrating. These two "types" are not interested in the same things and do not discuss them in the same way. In fact, long conversations are often difficult and frustrating for Sensors, as they would prefer to be experiencing and enjoying life, *as it is* in the moment. By contrast, Intuitives enjoy long conversations about possibilities and life *as it could be.* They are excited and energised by conversations like that. We can see then, that when a person wants to focus on individuation, it would be advantageous to be with a partner who experiences and converses about the world in a similar way. When we are with such a partner the chances are better that we will feel seen, understood, and supported.

In my relationship coaching practice and in my family medicine practice, I see this dynamic occurring time and time again. A person whose first intimate partner was their opposite, usually chooses a person whose personality type is very similar to their own the next time around. The second partner often shares three out of four letters, or preferences, represented in the Myers Briggs personality typing system. The good news is that out of the pain of dissolving that first relationship, one will be able to choose someone who is a more appropriate partner in the future.

I have found that, at midlife, the 6th *"C"* relationship factor becomes more significant when choosing a mate. In contrast to earlier in our lives, Sharing *Common Interests* assumes more importance as we approach retirement. At this stage of our lives, it makes sense to be with someone who likes the same type of music, books, and physical activity as we do. Later in life, intimate bonding is more about creating enjoyable companionship than it is about creating a home and a family together. Kingma attributes a long, harmonious union to a kind of camaraderie between partners:

> What forms the basis of a relationship that lasts is positive, loving feelings and the awareness that each of you have a whole complex of attributes that are of value

to the other and give pleasure to the other. These positive loving feelings are easily sustained when there is commonality. By commonality I mean there are a great many ideas, preferences, values, and perceptions that are held in common, as well as appropriately matched levels of physical and emotional energy...You will love, and have a happy life with the person whose looks, nature, habits, preferences, values and priorities call forth the truest expression of yourself, the person who invites you to blossom and grow. It is with this person that you truly have the potential of enjoying a relationship 'til death do you part.' (Kingma 136-138)

So, the relationship we are struggling with currently may not be in difficulty because either of us are *bad people* or because either of our characters is less than stellar. It may be ending because the developmental tasks of that relationship are complete and now we are experiencing significant differences in personality types and in preferences and interests that can't be reconciled. You see that each of you want to go in different directions; you may have different friends, entertain different retirement dreams, or may now hold different spiritual beliefs. You may want to spend your time differently and are struggling to find common ground other than your children, your house, and your retirement savings plans.

This struggle to find common ground, plus the inability to know what is going wrong, creates that gray feeling inside our souls. Once we begin to become consciously aware of what is going wrong for us, the grayness begins to lift as we gain insight. Then we have to seriously consider what to do. Can we make the marriage work through discussion and compromise, or is it time to move on?

Kingma identifies seven signs and symptoms that indicate a relationship is winding down. These things happen because it is so painful to tell ourselves the truth: our relationship is in trouble and may need to end (146-161).

1) Fights occur and re-occur, but do not reveal insights that have the effect of improving your relationship.

2) Irreconcilable differences develop. You develop different activities, habits, friends, values, and vacation preferences, so much so that very little common ground remains. Discussions and negotiations to try to reach joint compromise fail to find the comfortable middle ground.

3) Boredom develops that makes you feel listless, blue, disconnected, hopeless, or depressed. Your interactions don't provide sufficient pleasure for the relationship to flourish and feel healthy.

It is necessary to distinguish between boredom at work or within you personally--and boredom with your relationship. If you are bored with your life, and the relationship is good, then you can go to your spouse and discuss your feelings and come away feeling comforted and encouraged. As Tieger and Barron-Tieger's research shows, "those people most satisfied with their careers were also more satisfied in their relationships" (*Just Your Type* 313). It is crucial to take great care considering and identifying what aspect of your life you find boring. The following passage from Kingma's book comes from an individual who describes tedium--not with her job, her personal goals or her hobbies--but within her marriage:

> We weren't fighting. We didn't have money problems.
> Our sex life was functional, though not particularly
> exciting. Our house was pleasant enough and paid for.
> Our children were doing well enough in school--and yet I

found myself with the old is-that-all-there-is feeling most of the time. It was the sense that life would go on like this, unchanging, forever, that really depressed me, and I realized that I was in a marriage without any spark, and there hadn't been any for a long time. Even after seeing that, I wondered if it really was my marriage. So I looked at everything and everyone else in my life until I was satisfied that Phil and I didn't have anything in common anymore. When I saw that we really didn't, I knew then that it wasn't appropriate for us to be together any longer. I knew then that the end was in sight. From that point on I realized that there would be no going back. I didn't know how we would end or what would precipitate it, but I knew our relationship was over. (Kingma 151)

4) Emotional distance can develop out of the boredom you are feeling because you begin to reach out, not to your spouse, but to others for the emotional support you need. Most often, these essential emotional interactions are occurring with someone who is very similar to your personality type. Your spouse is no longer the person you go to first with something exciting or upsetting.

5) Changes in venue, for example moving to a new house or to a new city, can sometimes precipitate the collapse of a relationship. This is because one's home, neighbourhood, town, and friendships there support identity as a couple and as a family. When these known, familiar, comforting supports are removed, the relationship is put under stress and difficulties that formerly were hidden now come to the fore. Kingma reports that in her counselling, when one or the other partner is very uncomfortable about moving, this reticence can be an indicator that the relationship is coming to an end. Kingma says this dynamic is so

frequent an indicator of marital breakdown that she always takes it seriously (157).

6) Affairs are the first thing we think of as the sign that a marriage is about to end. Sometimes people engage in affairs to give themselves the nerve to end a marriage in which they have been struggling for a long time. Because sex is one of the main ways we distinguish friendship from a permanent love relationship, when someone has sex outside their relationship, it often becomes the deal-breaker. For many people, sex is the aspect of the marriage that makes it unique and exclusive; many of us take vows where we promise to have sex with our marriage partner only. Kingma says having sex outside the marriage is an unequivocal way to express a point. "That's one of the reasons why, when we are trying to end a relationship but don't know how, we often engage in an affair. Unconsciously, we know that the affair will communicate our real intentions--intentions which are still unfocussed or which we're afraid to express in a more direct way" (157-158).

7) Counseling or therapy sometimes occurs as a last resort when people reach the limit of their own problem-solving resources. Kingma says she finds couples often come in for counselling when one or the other partner feels that the relationship is over for them and they don't know how to tell their mate (160). Sometimes an individual subconsciously knows the relationship is over, but hasn't been able to be honest even with themselves-- the prospect of ending their relationship is that painful and terrifying. This frightening prospect may be able to be better faced in the safe context of couples' therapy, with the non-judgemental support of the counsellor's presence. Before we can examine our feelings, we first have to be able to acknowledge them. Then we can begin the process of ending the relationship as consciously as possible.

As you read through this list of signs indicative of the impending end of a relationship, did any of them ring true for you? If so, it is time to do some serious soul searching. If your relationship has already ended, becoming aware of these signs may provide insight into what was happening between the two of you, and what led up to your decision to end the relationship.

Telling the truth about what is going on within our relationship-- how we feel and what we are noticing--is difficult, yet necessary. Only when we tell the truth can we be set free to know what to do next. Maybe what we need to do is sit down for a gut-honest conversation with our partner, rather than continuing to drift along in grayness and denial. Maybe it's time for a personal retreat to pray for guidance and direction about our next step. Maybe it's time to find an experienced, wise, nonjudgmental counselor with whom to talk things over to help us to gain the crystal clear clarity we need before we proceed with that gut-honest talk. I believe wholeheartedly that telling *yourself* the truth about your deep unhappiness is the beginning of the process of discernment you must go through to decide what you want for your relationship. We must not deny that that there is a problem, and we must get ready to be gut-honest, transparent and vulnerable with ourselves, our intimate partner, and with a trusted counsellor.

As you tell yourself the truth about what you want for your particular relationship, it helps to look at relationships from the highest perspective possible. Overall, what do we need to make a relationship work? What is the most powerful possible perspective from which to view not only our intimate relationship, but all of our relationships? Is it really possible to become a master of relationship--to have relationships that are mostly healthy, happy, and whole, just as we desire to become individuals who are healthy, happy, and whole within ourselves?

I believe it is, and this is what I want to discuss in our closing chapter, *Empathy is the Key.*

CHAPTER SIX   Empathy Is the Key:
No Matter Where We Are in the Life of an Intimate Relationship
Empathy Is the Quality We Need

I had the privilege of interviewing a woman in my family practice a few days after her husband died. Over the years of seeing Olive and John, I observed them to be a loving, respectful, happily married couple. Olive and her husband were married at 18- and 20-years-old respectively. She came from a blue-collar family and had two siblings; he came from the same background but with ten siblings. When John died, they had been married 44 years.

I asked Olive how she would define marriage. *"It's being together in a partnership, with lots of winks and physical touch. It's doing what I can to make his day easier. And it's talking a lot, about everything--taking the time to really listen to what each other says."*

I then asked Olive what she saw as the biggest problem in today's marriages. *"It's me, me, me. Now, John and I belonged to the ' we' generation. Our main questions were, How can we make this work for us? How can I make my spouse's day easier? John would say things like, 'Hon, you look tired. Take a few minutes, and I'll make the salad.' ... When you get married, you get married! You have to want to be with each other. Even if I were going to a baby shower, he wanted to drive me over and then come and pick me up, so that he could be involved in some way in what I was doing. Marriage is a friendship. John was my best friend. We loved and we liked each other... I always made him number one, even above the kids. And he was willing to serve me, too. Material things were not our top priority. Although we struggled to make ends meet many times in our marriage, our relationship always came first."*

Olive is an ESTJ (Extroverted Sensing Thinking Judger). John was an ESFP (Extroverted Sensing Feeler Perceiver).

The two of them shared the same top *Love Language*: physical touch. Olive loved when John would wink at her across a crowded room. That wink said *you're my girl!* They loved cuddling up together on the couch watching a movie.

Olive said they never went to bed angry; they always cleared the air by talking a problem through.

Olive and John had two out of four personality type letters in common, which certainly helped. So did having a common top love language. But what this story illustrates for me is that they also were masters of a skill which, I believe, is absolutely necessary to a successful marriage--the skill of empathy.

Geoff Charley and Lucy Lidell in their booklet, *The Mirror Cards: A Powerful Tool to Enhance Your Relationship*, define empathy as being attuned to others in more than a superficial way.

> Empathy is the deep understanding we can have for other people. It springs from our ability to recognize ourselves in them--and them in us.
> Empathy is the bridge of the heart that spans the differences between people. It enables a two-way traffic of feelings and experiences, unrestricted by the 'border guards' of judgment and rejection. It links us to our partners through absolute acceptance of each other's realities. (Charley and Lidell 72)

After all is said and done, to thrive in an intimate relationship--to enjoy a healthy, close, long-term relationship--the quality most required is that of empathy extended from each partner to the other. We can attain this state after both partners have learned to know and accept *themselves*, and after they know and fully accept *the other*.

Author Jean Smith in *Now: The Art of Being Truly Present*, describes love in a way that combines the ideas of compassion, flexibility, and acceptance.

> Love--whether between life mates, parents and children, or friends--affirms the loved one for who he or she is. Our love relationships are not about changing another person to fit the ideal of 'love' our ego constructs, nor are they about rejecting other persons because, over time, they change, like everything else in life. Love is being truly present with the loyalty, caring and commitment that confirms the interconnectedness of all beings. (Smith 140)

In addition to empathy, we need to become curious and diligent students of our relationship, the *We* that we create, which is an entity unto itself and as real as each of us as individuals. We need to become as competent as possible at understanding how relationships work and at learning specific relationship skills if we are to commit and come successfully through the inevitable rocky patches along the path we agree to share. Empathy, compassion, kindness, and respect are the skills we need to understand and master in order to enjoy a successful relationship not only with an intimate partner, but with anyone.

When a couple stand in front of family and friends and say their vows, we get a shiver. Often, we feel like crying. At that moment, we have a sense of the profound nature of the vows they are speaking and of the monumental task they are undertaking.

Olive and John illustrated it beautifully in the mutual asking of a single question: *How can I make his or her day easier?* And they acted upon that question in the mutual doing of whatever it was that did, indeed, make their spouse's day easier. If each and every partnership were equally committed to an absolute acceptance of each other's realities--without judgement or rejection--and a willingness to see and do their best to make each other's day easier, this would go a long way toward creating healthy, harmonious relationships. Yes, intimacy requires conscious, intentional work in the sense that we need to make a continual, ongoing commitment to this way of seeing each other and seeing our relationship. But once the commitment is firmly made, we are on our way. Yes, we fail and recover, yet, once we ask for forgiveness and recommit to a mutual position of empathy, we can begin afresh.

For example, many couples I know have completely differing views on Christmas. For one partner, the Christmas season is something to endure, and for them Christmas day itself can seem like torture… all those people, all that noise, all those gifts, all that materialism! This is their perspective.

For that person's spouse, Christmas is the best time of the year... all that togetherness, all those decorations, all those traditions, all that great food! This person cannot see how anyone could view it any other way.

Many spouses have come to see how important Christmas is to their partners and they decide to stop resisting the holiday for the sake of their relationship. They come to realize that showing love means being willing to decorate the tree together, for example, and being willing to partake in the other traditions that the spouse holds dear because it means so much to them, and this, therefore, strengthens the relationship. This is the concept of empathy, practically applied. I believe that compassionate understanding of our mate and subsequent compassionate action are the elements that make a relationship work exceptionally well.

I think the most damaging concept regarding intimate partnership, and the hardest mental habit to break, is believing that there *is* such a person as a "magical other"--a person who can effortlessly see us, know us, and is willing and able to meet our every need (Hollis 79). After all, our fairy tales and romance novels say there is such a person. However, as we have learned, it appears that the "magical other" is a fiction and, in fact, we must come to realize that each of us must ultimately take responsibility for our own happiness, and that relationships require mutual conscious, intentional effort for fulfilment to occur.

I believe that the path to fulfilment in relationship is actually a perspective--a very powerful perspective--made up of three parts:

1) We agree to take responsibility to discover who we are, why we are here, and commit to acting in accordance with what we have discovered about ourselves. This creates inner fulfilment because we have discovered our own unique path.

2) We seek, with curiosity and non-judgment, to know our relationship partner, being willing to accept him or her as they truly are, with deep respect.

3) We become aware of our innate need for close relationships, and we take the responsibility to obtain the information and skills we need to interact well with those who are near and dear to us.

When we hold this three-part powerful perspective, we show respect for ourselves, for our partner, and for our relationship together. I believe this perspective will result in increased contentment in all of our relationships, and an increased sense of fulfilment and joy in our whole lives.

When I was asking people for their definitions of Soul Misery in Relationship, one response seemed more of an insightful summary statement about how to heal Soul Misery in Relationship.

"Simple and yet subtle different ways of communicating and viewing the world can cause a lot of pain in relationship. Unaddressed, what represents a little weed at first, can grow over time into a thorny garden. Then the underlying assumptions about each other become so strong that what your soul longs for in the other person to reflect back to you ultimately gets covered over and any attempt at weeding the garden only leaves you more hurt. However, the simple willingness to appreciate that others look at the world differently, and the humility not to turn your partner into a Pygmalion project (make them like you, in other words) allows love to flow and healing to begin. Then the weeds die of their own accord, and new plants representing more fun ways of being and relating to each other can be planted."

Yes, willingness to let go of assumptions + curiosity + non-judgement + empathy is a formula that can go a long way toward healing Soul Misery in Relationship, if both parties agree to approach their relationship in this way.

Most often in working with my relationship coaching clients, the couple come to the conclusion that they want to continue on as partners. But sometimes, despite their best efforts to grow as individuals and take full responsibility for themselves, plus their best effort to know and appreciate their spouse and to learn effective relationship tools, one or both partners may ultimately conclude that they want to dissolve their relationship. If this is the case, a conscious decision to come from the perspective of empathy will help their separation go as respectfully as possible. It is possible for a couple to transform their relationship from intimate partners to people who are friends--often co-parents--people who still respect and appreciate each other. This takes a lot of time, patience, talking, and usually someone to guide them through the process.

Likewise, one partner may have chosen to end the relationship, and later realize that if they had had the information they have now, they would not have needed to end it, or they could have tried applying some of the information or tools and that may have helped. This is a time to apply non-judgment to themselves, and kindness and empathy. I believe we are always doing the best we can under the circumstances. Sometimes we simply don't have the knowledge or the tools we need to do a job that needs doing. We can decide to love ourselves anyway! Then we can choose to learn from what we didn't know, embrace the personal growth that has occurred--even if it has been a painful experience--and carry on, willing to weave all of our experience into the fabric of the quilt that is our life.

Let us go forth, and using our new knowledge and tools, commit to the process of understanding ourselves and our partners, and to transforming ourselves and our relationships. Let us choose to love and accept ourselves as we are, love and accept others as they are, and embrace the life-long process of loving and learning in relationship.

Ability to influence	Endurance	Order
Achievement	Expertness	Passion
Advancement	Fairness	Peace
Adventure	Family	Philanthropy
Affection	Flexibility	Physical Challenge
Authenticity	Freedom	Personal Development
Beauty	Friendship	Play
Challenge	Generosity	Power
Change &Variety	Gentleness	Predictability
Comfort	Good Health	Recognition
Community	Happiness	Relaxation
Companionship	Helpfulness	Religious Belief
Competition	Honesty	Responsibility
Communication	Hopefulness	Risk
Conformity	Humour	Security
Connection	Independence	Self-respect
Contentment	Inner Harmony	Spirituality
Contribution	Integrity	Stability
Control	Involvement	Strength
Cooperation	Knowledge	Tradition
Courage	Leadership	Travel
Creativity	Love	Trust
Directness	Loyalty	Uniqueness
Economic Security	Mercy	Wealth
Elegance	Morality & Ethics	Wisdom

Accomplishment

Adaptability

Ambition

Athleticism

Authenticity

Cheerfulness

Commitment

Common Goals

Common Interests

Common Spiritual Beliefs

Companionship

Connection

Co-operation

Curiosity

Ease

Easy going nature

Emotional Health

Family Oriented

Fascinates Me

Financial Health

Flexibility

Fun

"Gets Me"

"Gives me Space"

Good Social Skills

Good With Kids

Harmony

Honesty

Humour

Independence

Integrity

Intelligence

Interests Me

Kindness

Knows & Accepts Me

Knows & Accepts Self

Likes Adventure

Likes Animals

Likes Kids

Likes the Outdoors

Likes to Read

Likes to Travel

Listening

Love

Loyalty

Magic

"My Equal"

Natural

Open-mindedness

Organization

Over His or Her "Ex"

Passion

Peacemaking

Physical Appearance

Physical Health

Positive Attitude

Reliability

Resilience

Respect

Same Cultural Background

Self-confidence

Sexual Chemistry

Sexual Fidelity

Simplicity

Soulfulness

Trust

Wants Kids

Wants to Live Where I Do

Work Ethic

- Barron-Tieger, Barbara and Paul Tieger. *Do What You Are.* New York: Little, Brown and Company, 1992.

This book helps us identify what our personality is in the Myers-Briggs personality typing system, and then gives us lots of information about that personality type. It is a wonderful starting place to discover the joys of knowing and living your unique personality type.

- Barron-Tieger, Barbara and Paul Tieger. *Just Your Type*. New York: Little, Brown and Company, 2000.

I found this book to be simply fascinating! It lists and describes the joys and the frustrations of all possible combinations of the 16 Myers-Briggs personality types. This book was designed to be used with marital relationships, but I have found that the information can be adapted to thinking about any relationship. I have used it to figure out why some relationships I am in seem to work so well and why others seem to struggle so much, using the lens of the Myers-Briggs way of looking at people.

- Barron- Tieger, Barbara and Paul Tieger. *The Art of Speed Reading People: How to Size People Up and Speak their Language.* New York: Little Brown and Company, 1998.

This is another fascinating book that explains how to quickly type a person using the Myers- Briggs personality typing system. The information about each type and temperament can give us greater insight into our partners, increasing our ability to extend compassion and empathy.

- Brown, Brené. *The Gifts of Imperfection.* Center City: Hazelden, 2010.

This is a wonderful book by a world renowned "shame" researcher. She introduces us to the term "midlife unravelling" and describes it with insight and compassion. She calls us to a life characterised by authenticity, self-compassion, gratitude, and joy.

- Briggs Myers, Isabel and Peter Myers. *Gifts Differing: Understanding Personality Type.* Mountain View: Consulting Psychologist's Press, 1995.

This classic bestseller of more than 250,000 copies explains in detail the Myers Briggs personality typing system. It gives us lots of tables that compare and contrast various aspects of type, and then discusses practical implications of type theory. It is very accessible and helpful for those who really want to understand people from the perspective of the Myers Briggs personality typing system.

- Chapman, Gary. *The Five Love Languages.* Chicago: Northfield Publishing, 1992.

This book explains that there are five different ways to express love in a relationship, helps us to discover which way is our way, and teaches us how to relate to a person whose language is different from ours. This concept is very practical and applicable to all of us, in all of our relationships. I have found that making people aware of the concept of the Five Love Languages, without exception, produces moments of fresh insight for them.

- Charley, Geoff, and Lucy Lidell. *The Mirror Cards: A Powerful Tool to Enhance Your Relationship.* London: Connections Book Publishing Ltd. 2003.

This deck of cards and accompanying booklet is used to bring clarity to relationships. Many times I have come to this deck of

cards, confused and unsure about a relationship I am in and--
working with the card I chose that day--come up with new ideas
and insights into what I could do to help strengthen or heal the
relationship.

- Gottman, John and Nan Silver. *The Seven Principles for Making Marriage Work.* New York: Three Rivers Press, 1999.

This is the most practical and helpful book I have read about how
marriage works. It also gives us practical, insightful advice about
how to improve one's marriage. The concept of the Four
Horsemen of the Apocalypse is introduced in this book.

- Hollis, James. *Finding Meaning in the Second Half of Life: How to Finally, Really Grow Up.* New York: Gotham Books, 2005.

I think Chapter Five, The Dynamics of Intimate Relationships, is
a must-read for all of us. We tend to think that if we could just
find our "magical other"--the one who sees us, knows us and
meets all our needs for us, all our misery in relationship would go
away. Dr Hollis explains that this is not so! We must each take
individual responsibility to meet our own deepest needs.
Becoming as whole as we can fits us to be the best possible
"other" when we enter an intimate relationship.

- Jeffers, Susan. *Feel the Fear and Do it Anyway.* New York: Ballantine Books, 2007.

The concept of the Whole Life Grid is found in this book. When
we realize that a whole life is made up of many aspects, not
simply our intimate relationships, we find an important key to
personal freedom and balance.

- Keirsey, David. *Please Understand Me II.* Del Mar: Prometheus Nemesis Book Company, 1998.

This book is utterly fascinating. Looking at people and relationships through the lens of temperament, this book is a wealth of information about how the different temperaments interact with one another. Studying this book yields much practical information that can be used to help us do better in our relationships.

- Kingma, Daphne. *Coming Apart: Why Relationships End and How to Live Through the Ending of Yours.* San Francisco: Conari Press, 2000.

Kingma believes that our primary reason to enter marriage-- which may be completely unconscious--is to complete individual developmental tasks. Therefore, when we have completed a particular developmental mission such as raising a family together, and we think our spouse cannot help us accomplish the next developmental task, we may not want to enter into that task with the same partner. I found the chapter "A Diagnostic Coda: When Love No Longer Works: Signs and Symptoms of Ending," particularly useful. This chapter outlines the seven signs that suggest a marriage may be about to end. Allowing ourselves to wonder if our marriage is still viable, nourishing, and sustainable is a very frightening prospect. Making yourself read this chapter may be scary, but it is very enlightening.

- Laney, Marti. *The Introvert Advantage.* New York: Workman Publishing, 2002.

This is the first book I have read that explains clearly what is positive about being an introvert. Most introverts have told me that they wish they were extraverts, as it is difficult to be in the minority. This book shows introverts how the world benefits by having them in it! The book is also good for extraverts who are in an intimate relationship with an introvert; it could help them understand things that may puzzle them about their partners. This is another book I recommend to almost every coaching client because it produces so many moments of fresh insight for virtually everyone who reads it.

- Moore, Thomas. *Original Self.* New York: Harper Collins, 2000.

This book speaks richly of what it takes to be a person of soul, someone who is able to relate to another person in the most mature way possible. I love the quote, attributed to Margaret Fuller, which he includes in his book. *"Union is only possible to those who are units."* This is something to aspire to!

- Moore, Thomas. *Soul Mates: Honouring the Mysteries of Love and Relationships.* New York: Harper Perennial, 1994.

This beautiful book is written by an "Idealist," (in Keirsey's temperaments system) for other Idealists. INFPs and INFJs in the Myers-Briggs personality system will "get" and love this book! Moore tells us that Soul Misery sufferers really need soul mates. This book explains what a soul mate is: someone who understands us deeply and who agrees to walk life's journey with us side-by-side.

- Nepo, Mark. *The Book of Awakening.* San Francisco: Conari Press, 2000.

This book of daily readings is simply wonderful! Nepo calls us to learn to love ourselves and others more deeply. He offers us a beautiful meditation at the conclusion of each day's reading. Especially helpful is the teaching he gives us about how to use our breath to help us be present to the difficult situations and emotions of our lives. Nepo had to face the prospect of dying from cancer. He came through this challenge determined to learn how to truly live!

- Osbon, Diane, *Reflections on the Art of Living: A Joseph Campbell Companion.* New York: HarperCollins, 1991.

This book is a collection of Joseph Campbell's wise and insightful quotations, as well as his thoughts about life's main themes. The concept of "the hero's journey" is introduced and discussed in this book.

- Quenk, Naomi. *Beside Ourselves.* Palo Alto: Davies-Black Publishing, 1993.

This book explains more about the intricacies of the Myers Briggs personality typing system. It is for someone who wants to understand it at the deepest levels, especially to understand the behaviour of each type, and most specifically the peculiar behaviour that doesn't seem to fit with that type. This happens when a person of any type is stressed. Fascinating!

- Rohr, Richard. *Falling Upwards.* San Francisco: Jossey Bass Publishing, 2011.

Richard Rohr is a Franciscan Monk who has thought a great deal about the two halves of life. He tells us that the first half is about creating "a container" for our lives and the second half should be dedicated to exploring the contents of the container. When we enter the midlife transition period, the way we look at God, work, nature, and relationships can change and this can take us by surprise. Rohr does a masterful job of helping us make sense of these changes in our thinking.

- Ruiz, Don Miguel. *The Four Agreements.* San Rafael: Amber-Allen Publishing, 1997.

For me, the second agreement, "Don't Take Things Personally," and the third agreement, "Don't Make Assumptions," are powerful precepts that have the potential to make relationships better between any two human beings. In his book, Ruiz explained these two agreements so clearly and simply that I could see right away how to apply them to any and all of my relationships. Doing so offers the potential for more peace and contentment.

- Ruiz, Don Miguel. *The Mastery of Love*. San Rafael: Amber-Allen Publishing, 1999.

In this book Ruiz explains how and why we wound each other in relationship, and then in simple and beautiful, clear terms, he explains how we can learn to be non-judgmental and helpful to others. My favourite chapters are five, The Perfect Relationship, and six, The Magic Kitchen. I recommend both *The Four Agreements* and *The Mastery of Love* to all clients I coach who are experiencing either personal Soul Misery or Soul Misery in Intimate Relationship.

- Sher, Barbara. *Wishcraft*. New York: Viking Press, 1979.

Barbara Sher has been called the "godmother" of life coaching. I discovered her book after I had finished writing *Healing Soul Misery: Finding the Pathway Home*. I was amazed to find that way back in 1979, Sher clearly described the same process that-- 18 years later--Don Miguel Ruiz called "domestication" in his book, *The Four Agreements*.

Sher tells us that to get what we want, we must first know what we want. She explains that many of us are hard-working, responsible people who know *how* to get things done, but have never felt free to explore *what* we actually *want* to do. She tells us that what we want is not a luxury that can wait until we have taken care of all the "serious" business of life. It is a necessity. *"What we want is what we need."* (Sher, xx-xxiii).

Her book is divided in two. The first section is devoted to helping us know who we are and what we want. The second section gives us practical tools to get what we want. The first section is the "Wish" section; the second is the "Craft" section!

By 2009, thirty years after the book was first published, it had sold 650,000 copies! I highly recommend doing the exercises she gives us in the book, as without exception, they have helped my coaching clients and myself get clear on what we want and need to feel that our lives are truly satisfying.

- Smith, Jean. *Now: The Art of Being Truly Present.* Somerville: Wisdom Publications, 2004.

This is a beautiful and inspiring book of short reflections written from the Buddhist perspective on topics such as breath, grief, and love. My favourite definition of love comes from the latter section: "Love is being truly present with the loyalty, caring and commitment that confirms the interconnectedness of all beings."(140) Beautiful, isn't it?

- Tieger , Paul and Barbara Barron Tieger. *Nurture by Nature.* New York: Little, Brown and Company, 1997.

This book makes the case for raising our children by trying to recognize their personality type early and then nurturing children according to the unique requirements of their type. Tieger and Barron-Tieger teach us how to determine a child's personality type, then they give specific tips for each of them, tied to the age group of the child: preschool, school-aged, and adolescence.

- Wagele, Elizabeth. *The Happy Introvert: A Wild and Crazy Guide for Celebrating Your True Self.* Berkeley: Ulysses Press, 2006.

This upbeat, funny book helps introverts embrace who they are. It is packed with practical, common-sense information that is helpful for helping the introvert understand and nurture themselves, as well as helping the introvert do better in their relationships. This book made me laugh and cheered me up!

- Whyte, David. *The Three Marriages: Reimagining Work, Self and Relationship.* New York: Riverhead Books, 2009.

David Whyte looks at life and marriage in a very wry, eyes-open way. I laughed out loud on several occasions while reading his wonderful book. Here is an example of one of his perceptive insights:

> Marriage is where we realize that the other person actually is alive and has notions and desires that have very little to do with our own hopes and dreams.... Marriage is where we realize that we have married a stranger whom we must get to know... Marriage is where all of these difficult revelations can consign us to imprisonment or help us become larger, more generous, more amusing, more animated participants in the human drama. (263)

How perceptive! How inspiring!

BIBLIOGRAPHY

Barron-Tieger, Barbara and Paul Tieger. *Just Your Type*. New York: Little, Brown and Company, 2000. Print.

Brown, Brené. *The Gifts of Imperfection*. Center City, Minnesota: Hazelden, 2010. Print.

Briggs Myers, Isabel and Peter Myers. *Gifts Differing: Understanding Personality Type*. Mountain View: Consulting Psychologist's Press, 1980. Print.

Brittin, David. "Change and Wonder: *A Butterfly Complete Metamorphosis*." Vimeo, 29 Oct. 2009. Web. 01 Aug. 2013. (www.vimeo.com/7203408).

Chapman, Dr. Gary. *The Five Love Languages*. Chicago: Northfield Publishing, 1992. Print.

Charley, Geoff and Lucy Lidell. *The Mirror Cards: A Powerful Tool to Enhance Your Relationship*. London: Connections Book Publishing Ltd., 2003. Print.

Gleeson, Susan. *Healing Soul Misery: Finding the Pathway Home*. Lulu.com. 2011. Print

Gottman, John. *The Seven Principles for Making Marriage Work*. New York: Three Rivers Press, 1999. Print.

Hollis, James. *Finding Meaning in the Second Half of Life: How to Finally Really Grow Up.* New York: Penguin Group, 2005. Print.

Jeffers, Susan. *Feel the Fear and Do it Anyway.* New York: Ballantine Books, 2007. Print.

Keirsey, David. *Please Understand Me II.* Del Mar: Prometheus Nemesis Books, 1998. Print.

Kingma, Daphne. *Coming Apart.* San Francisco: Conari Press, 2000. Print.

Mindell, Arnold. *Dreaming While Awake: Techniques for 24-Hour Lucid Dreaming.* Charlottesville: Hampton Roads Publishing Company, 2000. Print.

Moore, Thomas. *Original Self.* New York: HarperCollins, 2000. Print.

New International Version Bible. Grand Rapids: Zondervan Publishing House, 1994. Print.

O'Donohue, John. *Anam Cara.* New York: Harper Collins Books, 1997. Print.

Osbon, Diane. *Reflections on the Art of Living: A Joseph Campbell Companion.* New York: HarperCollins, 1992. Print.

Ruiz, Miguel. *The Four Agreements.* San Rafael: Amber Allen Publishing, 1997. Print.

Sher, Barbara. *Wishcraft*. New York: Ballantine Books, 1979. Print.

Smith, Jean. *Now: The Art of Being Truly Present.* Maine: Wisdom Publications, 2004. Print.

Tieger, Paul and Barbara Barron-Tieger. *Do What You Are.* New York: Little, Brown and Company, 2000. Print.

Tieger, Paul and Barbara Barron-Tieger. *Nurture by Nature.* New York: Little, Brown and Company, 1997. Print.

Whyte, David. *The Three Marriages: Reimagining Work, Self and Relationship.* New York: Riverhead Books, 2009. Print.

ABOUT THE AUTHOR

Susan Gleeson attained her medical degree from Queen's University in Kingston, Ontario, in 1979. She completed her family medicine residency at Queen's two years later. Susan went on to complete a Masters of Science in Community Health and Epidemiology, also at Queen's. She has now practised family medicine for over 30 years. Wanting to broaden her ability to heal, Susan became a certified life coach through the Coaches Training Institute; in 2006 she completed their Organization and Relationship Systems Coaching Program. Three years later, Susan completed the Coaches Training Institute Co-Active Leadership program. She also experienced the Bigger Game workshop led by Rick Tamlyn, and in 2010, became a Bigger Game facilitator.

Susan became interested in the expressive arts, and in particular began to explore acrylic and watercolour painting at the Haliburton School of the Arts. She discovered the Expressive Arts program there, a program to enable professionals such as social workers, ministers, teachers, doctors and nurses to integrate the expressive arts into their work. Susan received her Ontario College Graduate Certificate in the Expressive Arts in 2013. Along the way she discovered Nia, a cardiovascular exercise program that incorporates music and expressive movement. Susan has become a certified Nia 5 Stages Instructor and a Nia Blue Belt Instructor.

As a family physician, life coach, and expressive arts practitioner, Susan was privileged to observe many close personal relationships in action. She became fascinated by the inner workings of intimate relationships, began to study them extensively and--based on her learning and observation--was led to write *If I Love You, Why Is It So Hard to Live With You?*

Susan also wrote *Healing Soul Misery: Finding the Pathway Home,* which she self-published in 2011. To learn more, visit www.healingsoulmisery.com.